D. Pathomvanich · K. Imagawa (eds.)

Hair Restoration Surgery in Asians

D. Pathomvanich · K. Imagawa
Editors

Hair Restoration Surgery in Asians

Springer

Editors
Damkerng Pathomvanich, MD, FACS, ABHRS
DHT Clinic, private practice, Bangkok, Thailand
Consulting Staff at Bumrungrad Hospital, Bangkok
General Hospital and Vichaiyuth Hospital Director
Fellowship Training Program in Hair Restoration Surgery (ISHRS) since 2003

Kenichiro Imagawa, MD, PhD, ABHRS
Medical Director, private practice, Yokobi Clinic, Yokohama, Japan
Board of Governor of the Japan Society of Aesthetic and Reconstructive Surgery
Program Director of ISHRS Regional Workshop Asian Hair Surgery 2007

ISBN 978-4-431-54726-6 ISBN 978-4-431-99659-0 (eBook)
DOI 10.1007/978-4-431-99659-0
Springer Tokyo Berlin Heidelberg New York

Softcover re-print of the Hardcover 1st edition 2010

Printed on acid-free paper

Springer is a part of Springer Science+Business Media (www.springer.com)

Foreword

Why a new book on hair restoration surgery?

The answer is simple: people of Asian physical characteristics make up approximately 60% of this planet's population. The proportion is even greater if we include some of those from Oceania and the native races of North and South America who carry a large proportion of Asian genes.

Asians are a genetically diverse group of people who may be subdivided into at least 30 distinct subgroups with varying physical characteristics and hair types. Their hair varies from the coarse, but relatively sparse, hair of the Japanese and Han Chinese to the fine, densely packed, and wavy hair seen in people from some parts of India. Baldness also varies from the minimal degrees seen in south Asia to the very severe grades commonly seen on the subcontinent. There is also considerable variation within each ethnic group, as within the Caucasian population.

The surgical transplantation of autografts of human hair was first described in detail in a series of articles by Dr. Shoji Okuda in Japan in 1939 [1]. In his articles he alluded to prior work on hair implantation and autotransplantation done by several other researchers. Okuda's technique was used for the replacement of eyebrows and pubic and axillary hair, but scalp hair was never mentioned. This omission does not mean that scalp hair transplantation was not done at all, only that it was not listed as a target site in the various published articles. The use of surgical skills for the restoration of lost scalp hair was probably regarded as a purely frivolous procedure in very conservative pre-war Japan. Mention of such "cosmetic" procedures may have been deliberately omitted or edited from the text of articles submitted for publication in the very conservative medical journals of the day [2].

With the disruption caused by the war, hair transplantation was ignored in Asia for decades and was "rediscovered" by the New York dermatologist Norman Orentreich in 1959 [3]. At the time he was investigating whether skin with certain dermatological conditions exhibited donor or recipient dominance when transplanted from one site to another. Male baldness appeared to be a condition that exhibited donor dominance [4].

Surgical hair restoration was taken up only slowly by doctors in Asia after WW II, although it was evident from the popularity of hairpieces that Asians disliked baldness as much as their Western counterparts. The implantation of artificial hair was developed in Japan from 1964 as an alternative to hairpieces and enjoys a considerable market share in that country to the present day [5].

Rapid improvements in hair transplant technique occurred in the West from the mid-1970s onward. The motivating factor was the establishment, by the late American dermatologist D. Bluford Stough, of a series of scientific meetings to discuss hair transplantation. Almost concurrently, a textbook on the subject was published by fellow dermatologist Dr. O'Tar T. Norwood of Oklahoma City [6]. Several other textbooks by dermatologists and plastic surgeons followed in the decade ahead. A quantum leap occurred with the establishment of a bimonthly newsletter on hair transplantation by Dr. Norwood in 1990 [7]. For the rapid exchange of ideas and techniques, this medium proved far superior to the conventional surgery and dermatology journals, and even the meetings of the day, which were often restricted to members of certain specialty groups.

The next important step was the formation of a society open to all physicians interested in surgical hair replacement. This group was initiated by Dr. Dowling Stough, (son of the above-mentioned Bluford Stough) and actively supported by Dr. Norwood and many others [8].

With a bimonthly newsletter and an annual scientific meeting, hair restoration surgery was in the fast lane at last, and improvements have been numerous and impressive. As with any new field, there were many false starts and "dead-ends" over the subsequent years, but we have now achieved ways to efficiently perform the single hair procedures described as the ideal by Dr. Hajimi Tamura of Japan in 1943 [9].

With the rapidly increasing wealth and sophistication of Asian people and their willingness to embrace cosmetic surgery procedures, it is imperative that they have a book reflecting their specific requirements. Hopefully this is such a book, and I wish the editors and contributors every success with this important publication.

Richard C. Shiell, MBBS
Hair Transplant Surgeon, Melbourne, Australia

About the Author:

Dr. Shiell was co-author of the second edition of *Hair Transplant Surgery* along with Dr. O.T. Norwood in 1984 and has contributed chapters to many other books. He has authored many scientific papers, has been a prolific contributor to the specialty newsletter *Hair Transplant Forum*, and was its editor from 1996 to 1998.

Dr. Shiell was the Foundation President of the Australian Society of Hair Transplant Surgeons in 1984 and a Foundation Member of the International Society of Hair Restoration Surgery in 1993. In 1997, in Barcelona, he received the International Society's Golden Follicle Award for Services to the Profession and in 1999, in San Francisco, the society presented him with its highest honor, the Manfred Lucas Award.

Now retired from active practice, Dr. Shiell was a Foundation Member of the American Board of Hair Restoration Surgery, the Australian College of Cosmetic Surgery, and is a past-president of the Australasian Hair and Wool Research Society.

References

1. Okuda S (1939) Clinical and experimental studies on hair transplanting of living hair. Jpn J Dermatol Urol 46:537–587 (in Japanese)
2. Senior members of the profession today recall similar attitudes still prevailing in Western society when they started performing hair transplantation (HT) in the 1960s and 1970s.
3. Orentreich N (1959) Autografts in alopecias and other selected dermatological conditions. Ann N Y Acad Sci 83:463–479
4. This theory was challenged many years later by Prof. J.C. Kim of South Korea in 1994, and his work was later supported by his countryman, Dr. Sungjoo Hwang, in 2006. Both showed that the recipient site does exert some influence on long-term results. In retrospect, Dr. Okuda 60 years earlier had said, when speaking of the vigorous growth of transplanted eyebrow hairs, "later they gradually assimilate the recipient graft area morphology."
5. Yamada S, Fukuta K(1996) Synthetic hair grafting. In: Stough DB, Haber RS (eds) Hair replacement: surgical and medical. Mosby Year-Book, St. Louis, pp 345–357
6. Norwood OT (1973) Hair transplant surgery. Thomas, Springfield
7. Hair Transplant Forum International
8. The International Society for Hair Restoration Surgery was founded in Dallas, Texas, in 1993.
9. Tamura H (1943) Concerning hair transplantation (2nd report). Jpn J Dermatol Venereol 53:76 (in Japanese)

Preface

Hair transplantation as we know originated in Japan [1]. However, the art and science of hair transplantation have received further progression and refinement in Western countries [2]. Because the outcome of hair transplantation today is more natural, and good density can be achieved in just one or two sessions compared to the several sessions required in the past, hair transplantation is in demand worldwide. With an influx of new physicians entering this challenging field of medicine, we believe that further education and training are imperative and must be available to provide a standard of medical practice.

A recent survey conducted by the International Society for Hair Restoration Surgery (ISHRS) reported that 57 542 procedures were performed in Asian countries in 2006, a significant rise from 20 673 in the year 2005 [3]. However, the number is still very low compared with North America and Europe. We believe Asian hair is different from that of Caucasians, and not all aspects of the procedures used for Caucasians are applicable to Asian patients and their Asian hair.

There are many hair transplantation textbooks available for hair restoration surgeons; however, each text contributes only a few pages pertinent to hair restoration in Asians. So, we felt there is a need for a text exclusively devoted to Asian hair. We believe this might be the first textbook dedicated to the many aspects of hair restoration surgery in Asians.

The text carries several objectives. For beginners, it provides a simple explanation of hair restoration surgery. For experienced surgeons, it serves as a quick reference. Globalization increases the possibility that surgeons working in the West may be approached by Asians for hair transplantation. Although not an encyclopedia of hair restoration, this text still provides a quick and complete reference on Asian hair and the differences in the patients' demands. We try to provide practical tips. Chapters on regional transplantation such as eyebrows, eyelashes, sideburns, beards, and mustaches are incorporated in addition to the usual scalp hair restoration. We tried our best to organize this book with a limited number of pages and illustrations but still give all readers complete knowledge of Asian hair restoration surgery.

The editors initially considered the compilation of the experience of all hair transplant surgeons working in Asia. This, however, is a difficult task to initiate. During the Regional ISHRS Live Surgery Workshop in Yokohama, Japan, the authors met and all agreed to limit the number of contributors. We were fortunate that all the authors we approached agreed to write on their specialized fields, sharing experience from their decades of practice.

Every valuable contribution to hair restoration surgery is ultimately a contribution to restoration of confidence for the patient. This compilation is an attempt to pursue the same noble goal.

Damkerng Pathomvanich, MD, FACS
Kenichiro Imagawa, MD, PhD

References

1. Okuda S (1939) Clinical and experimental studies on hair transplanting of living hair (in Japanese). Jpn J Dematol Urol 46:537–587
2. Orentreich N (1959) Autografts in alopecia and other selected dermatological conditions. Ann N Y Acad Sci 83:463–479
3. International Society of Hair Restoration Surgery (2007) Practice census results. ISHRS, Tokyo

Acknowledgments

Words of acknowledgment are far from sufficient to express my gratitude to every one of my colleagues for their invaluable efforts to bring about this text. The deepest of my gratitude however is reserved for Dr. Richard C. Shiell, who readily accepted my request for the laborious task of editing the text. He has been the strongest support in bringing the team from different directions to work together. His advice was valuable to all the authors, and his patience and friendliness made me feel at ease and without stress.

My parents and my family have been with me through every endeavor. The very thought of writing a book was given unabated support, as ever. This task would not have been possible without their help.

To obtain an ideal publisher was not an easy task because there are a limited number of physicians worldwide who are doing hair restoration surgery compared with other fields of medicine. I would like to express my sincere thanks to our publisher, Springer, and to Mrs. Kambara for making the impossible mission possible.

Last, but not least, I thank Drs. Richard Shiell, Jerry Wong, Jung-Chul Kim, Kitaro Ohmori, Sungjoo Tommy Hwang, Kristine S. Bunagan, Bertram Ng, Konqkiat Laorwong, Radha R. Palakurthi, Ms. Patcharee, and Ms. Saranya for their contributions to the chapters.

This book might have been delayed as much as a year without the help of Bertram Ng, a rising star in our field of hair restoration surgery. His valuable time was well spent in double-checking the grammar and organizing the chapters before sending them to Dr. Richard Shiell for further editing. His participation in bringing out this contemporary is deeply appreciated.

Damkerng Pathomvanich, MD, FACS

Contents

Contributors

Kulakarn Amonpattana, MD
Plastic surgeon, private practice, Bangkok, Thailand
Graduate Fellow DHT Clinic, ISHRS

Mary Jo Kristine S. Bunagan, MD, DPDS
Consultant dermatologist, Department of Dermatology,
Davao Medical Center, Philippines
Fellow in Hair Restoration Surgery DHT Clinic, ISHRS

Sungjoo "Tommy" Hwang, MD, PhD, ABHRS
Dermatologist, private practice, Korea
Board of Directors, American Board of Hair Restoration Surgery

Kenichiro Imagawa, MD, PhD, ABHRS
Medical Director, private practice, Yokobi Clinic, Yokohama, Japan
Board of Governor, Japan Society of Aesthetic and Reconstructive Surgery

Jung-Chul Kim, MD, PhD
Director of Hair Transplantation Center, Kyungpook National University Hospital
Professor of Department of Immunology, School of Medicine,
Kyungpook National University, Daegu, Korea

Kongkiat Laorwong, MD
Consultant, Bangkok Phuket Hospital
Medical Director, private practice, Absolute Hair Clinic, Phuket, Thailand

Bertram Ng, MBBS
Hair Transplant Surgeon, private practice, Hong Kong
Fellow in Hair Restoration Surgery, DHT Clinic, ISHRS

Kitaro Ohmori, MD, PhD
Emeritus Director of Clinica Ichigaya, Tokyo, Japan
Exective Director, Japan Society of Aesthetic and Reconstructive Surgery

Radha R. Palakurthi, MBBS, DD
Dermatologist and Hair Transplant Surgeon, private practice, India
Fellow in Hair Restoration Surgery, DHT Clinic, ISHRS

Patcharee Thienthaworn
Registered Nurse, DHT Clinic Bangkok, Thailand

Damkerng Pathomvanich, MD, FACS, ABHRS
DHT Clinic, private practice, Bangkok, Thailand
Consulting Staff at Bumrungrad Hospital, Bangkok
General Hospital and Vichaiyuth Hospital Director,
Fellowship Training Program in Hair Restoration Surgery (ISHRS) since 2003

Sarunya Manochai
DHT Clinic, registered Nurse, Bangkok, Thailand

Jerry Wong, MD, ABHRS
Hassan & Wong Hair Transplant Center, private practice, Vancouver, Canada

Part I
History and the Past

Back to the Future: A Brief but Significant History of Hair Transplantation in Asians

K. Imagawa

Orentreich has been honored as the father of hair transplantation. However, one should realize that some Japanese pioneers had done great work in hair transplantation even before the release of Orentreich's papers in 1959 [1].

Shoji Okuda (1886–1962) is the best known among these pioneers. He published five series of articles titled "Clinical and experimental study of living hair transplantation" in the *Japanese Journal of Dermatology* in 1939, reporting 200 cases of reconstruction in cicatricial and congenital alopecia of the scalp as well as pubic atrichia [2]. His techniques employed specifically designed "round saws" 1.0–5.0 mm in diameter that closely resembled Orentreich's finger-operated round punches. In the Okuda papers we can find almost everything relevant to modern hair transplantation, including the principle of "donor dominance" and the miserable results of hetero-transplantation of human hair. Unfortunately, Okuda did not mention male pattern hair loss (MPHL) as a treatable condition, and thus Dr. Orentreich is honored as the first to use these innovative techniques for MPHL.

Because of the chaos of World War II, his papers drew little attention for some time. Nevertheless, his techniques have been spotlighted again and termed the "Okuda/Orentreich technique" by a German doctor, H.C. Friedrich, who discovered Okuda's work and thesis in his German-translated abstracts [3]. Because the Okuda papers were written in old *kanji* (old pictographs) and the writing was often unintelligible, even Japanese found it difficult to understand his writings until the complete English version translated by Yoshihiro Imagawa appeared in 2003 [4].

Mysteriously, no information about Okuda himself could be obtained until Inui and Itami made a thorough search in 2008. They discovered Okuda's curriculum vitae and license number on the list of medical licenses in 1930 and succeeded in tracing his family. According to an interview with his grandson, Dr. Takaaki Okuda, Shoji Okuda was born in 1886 in Nara and passed the Medical Practitioners Qualifying Examination in 1912 through self-education and training at Mitsui Charity Hospital and Juntendo Hospital. He started his practice as a general practitioner but later specialized in ophthalmology. He received his doctorate from Osaka University in 1941, worked from home for a long time, and passed away at the age of 77 [5] (Fig. 1). He would not have heard of the developments in the science of hair transplantation in the United States and elsewhere.

D. Pathomvanich and K. Imagawa (eds.), *Hair Restoration Surgery in Asians*
DOI 10.1007/978-4-431-99659-0_1, © Springer 2010

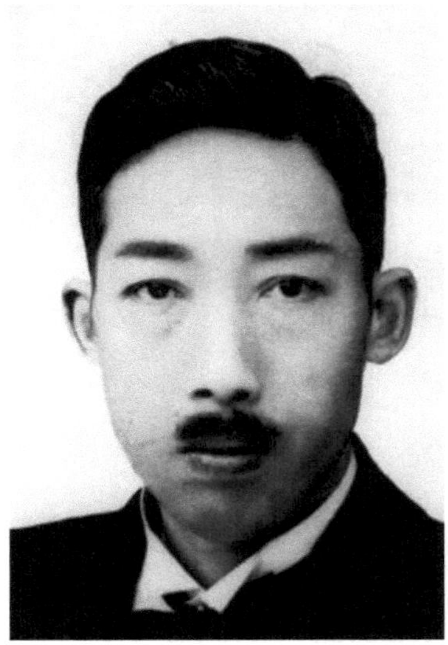

Fig. 1. Dr. Shoji Okuda (photograph courtesy of Dr. Takaaki Okuda)

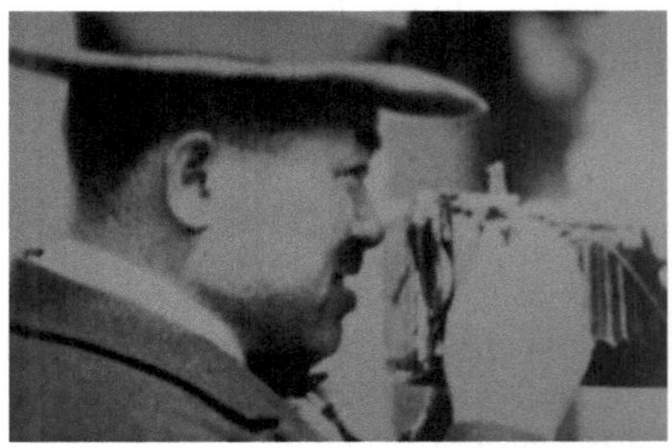

Fig. 2. Dr. Masao Sasakawa (from *Kyudeikai-Kaishi* 1928, volume 32)

In 1929, Masao Sasakawa (1887–1932), while he was Professor of Dermatology at Keio University, reported the results of a 10-month follow-up of cases in which doubled-up human hairs were inserted in the subcutaneous tissue of cicatricial alopecia and alopecia totalis using a special needle [6]. Shiell pointed out that this was a very insightful approach as artificial hair implantation using synthetic hair was very popular in Japan from the late 1970s until the present time [7] (Fig. 2).

Hajime Tamura (1897–1977) performed many hair transplant procedures when he was Professor of Urology at Tokyo Women's Medical University. It was reported that 127 cases in 1937 failed but that 136 cases after 1939 showed good results [8]. His techniques using single-hair grafts produced an excellent natural appearance. However, he seems to have lost interest in hair restoration after he became Professor of Urology at Keio University in 1944 (Fig. 3). Had doctors in Western countries become aware of his achievements earlier and adopted his techniques, the history of hair transplantation would have taken a different course and punch grafting may not have become the standard procedure for more than 30 years.

Fig. 3. Dr. Hajime Tamura (from Issui Nikki, 1978)

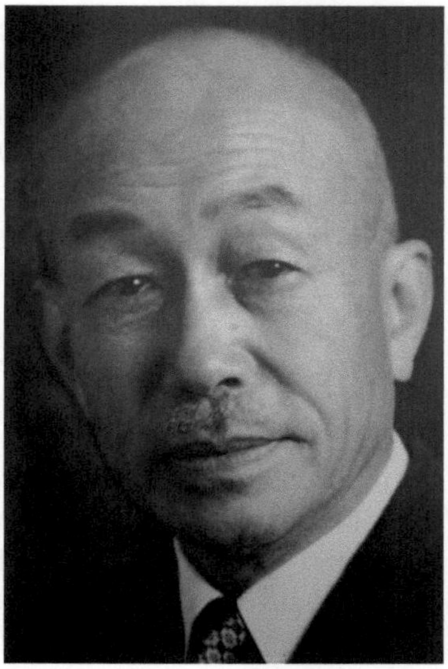

Fig. 4. Dr. Keiichi Fujita (from *Journal of Japan Society of Aesthetic Surgery* 1985, volume 24-1)

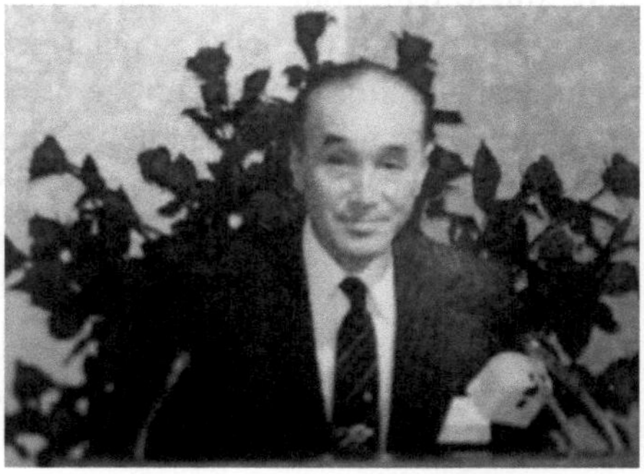

Keiichi Fujita graduated from Tokyo University in 1947. While he worked for Tama Zensei Yen in the Institute of Hansen Disease, he performed many eyebrow reconstructions using single-hair grafts. Fujita reported that scalp hair transplanted as eyebrows grew long but behaved more like eyebrow hair after 1 year. This phenomenon was later known as "recipient influence" [9]. Also, he reported that donor hairs would grow even when kept in refrigeration for 4 days [10]. No further reports were released in regard to hair restoration after he was appointed Professor at the Japanese Army Medical Hospital and Medical University in 1957. I wonder whether he might have grown tired of the long hours of tedious work (Fig. 4). Late in the lives of Tamura and Fujita, the Okuda/Orentreich techniques had gained popularity in Western countries. I wonder whether they knew and, if so, how they felt about it.

After that there were no more reports of surgeons using single-hair grafts in Asian countries until Choi and Kim reported their attempts at using small grafts in 1992 [11,12]. Mr. Paek was using single hairs to restore leprosy-affected patients well before this time, however, and he was presented with an award by the

International Society of Hair Restoration Surgery (ISHRS) at their annual meeting in Hawaii 2000 for his long-unreported contribution to our field [13]. Western surgeons such as Uebel, Unger, and Shiell were also using single hairs cut from the sides of plugs to soften the front edge. These cases were mentioned at meetings but were not published in the literature until Emmanuel Marritt's paper in the very early 1980s [14] and the textbook by Norwood and Shiell in 1984 [15].

Two Techniques of Hair Transplantation in Asia

Until the end of the 1980s, macrografts had been overwhelmingly made of artificial fibers because of the aggressive marketing of the latter as "natural-looking implants." When the author first started hair practice in the late 1980s, many colleagues mistook hair transplantation as artificial fiber implantation.

The widespread acceptance of hair transplantation in Asia owed a great deal to Drs. Choi and Kim, who invented an epoch-making implanter. Initially, they used only single-hair grafts and later two- and three- "bundle hair" grafts, which are synonymous with the more standardized term "follicular units" (FUs). Follicular unit transplantation (FUT) and the use of Choi or KNU implanters have characterized the two standard techniques used in Korea and Japan up to the present time. Very few Asian doctors adopted Western techniques of hair restoration until the early 1990s.

Other Techniques of Hair Restoration in Asia

Alopecia reduction has never been popular because the Asian scalp is comparatively tight. The maximum amount of bald skin that can be removed is less, and the pain increases dramatically with each additional millimeter (mm) past the optimum level of laxity when Asian surgeons try to remove the same width of scalp as described in the Western literature. Also, the scar in the thinning area becomes wider and more noticeable and there are many other potential complications, such as stretch-back, stretch-atrophy, and slots. Although a few doctors still offer this procedure, the numbers have markedly declined.

In contrast, scalp flaps were very popular in Japan. Many Japanese plastic surgeons were convinced that scalp flaps work better than grafts for the black, coarse, and straight Asian hair. This method is, however, not without its complications as the high incidence of smoking in Asians and their tight scalps would increase the potential risks of telogen effluvium, flap necrosis, and hair loss in the area from where the flap was taken. With the rapid progression of FU transplantation, however, the use of flaps in both MPHL and female pattern hair loss (FPHL) has decreased (see the chapter "Is There a Place for the Scalp Flap in Modern Hair Restoration Surgery?" in this volume).

References

1. Orentreich N (1959) Autografts in alopecia and other selected dermatological conditions. Ann N Y Acad Sci 83:463–479
2. Okuda S (1939) Clinical and experimental studies on hair transplanting of living hair. Jpn J Dematol Urol 46:537–587 (in Japanese)
3. Friederich HC (1970) Indikation und Technik der Operativ-plastischen Behandlung des Haaeverlustes. Hauturzt 21:197–202 (in German)
4. Shiell RC (2004) The Okuda papers. Hair Transplant Forum Int 14:1–6
5. Inui S, Itami S (2009) Personal communication (paper submitted)
6. Sasakawa M (1930) Concerning hair transplantation. Jpn J Dermatol Urol 30:76 (in Japanese)
7. Shiell RC (2004) Tamura, Sasakawa and Fujita now translated. Hair Transplant Forum Int 14:41–46
8. Tamura H (1943) Concerning hair transplantation (2nd report). Jpn J Dermatol Urol 53:76 (in Japanese)
9. Fujita K (1953) Brow plasty. Lepra 22:218 (in Japanese)
10. Fujita K (1954) Homologous punctiform living hair graft. Lepra 23:364 (in Japanese)
11. Uebel CO (1991) Micrografts and minigrafts: a new approach to baldness surgery. Ann Plast Surg 27:476–482
12. Choi YC, Kim JC (1992) Single hair transplantation using the Choi Hair Transplanter. Dermtol Surg Oncol 18:945–948
13. Ahn SY (2000) We salute you, Mr. Paek. Hair Transplant Forum Int 10:151
14. Marritt E (1980) Transplantation of single hairs from the scalp as eyelashes. J Dermatol Surg Oncol 6:271–273
15. Norwood O, Shiell RC (1984) Hair transplant surgery. Thomas, Springfield

Part II
Asian Hair: Knowing the Differences

The Prevalence of Male Pattern Baldness in Asian Men

R. Palakurthi

The prevalence of male pattern baldness (MPB) in Caucasians is well documented by Norwood [1] and Hamilton [2]. Takashima, Iju, and Sudo [3] and Kakizo [4] studied MPB in Japanese and found that it was minimal before the age of 40 and, although incidence increased with age, it was lower than in Caucasians.

In Singapore, P.H. Tang et al. [5] reported a prevalence of 63% in Norwood type I to VII. The prevalence increased with age from 32% among young adults aged between 17 and 26 years to almost 100% for those in their eighties.

In Bangkok, Thailand, D. Pathomvanich conducted a randomized study in 1997 including 1124 Asian men (local Thai and Chinese) between the ages of 18 and 90 [6]. The prevalence of baldness was reported as 38.52%; this alarmingly high figure approached that of Caucasians, rather than the one-fourth to one-third reported in previous studies [3]. Also as seen in Caucasians, the prevalence increased with age, affecting 11% young adults aged over 20 years and reaching 61.78% at 70 years of age. The results compared to the Norwood and Hamilton groups are summarized in Figs. 1 and 2. There were, however, two limitations in this survey. First, the small number of men over 80 years (31 men) might have biased results when compared to the Norwood study in the same age group. Also, there were two Asian subgroups involved in this study, Thai and Chinese.

In China, a population-based cross-sectional study of 3519 Chinese men in July 2008 reported a prevalence of 19.9% of MPB [7]. The prevalence increased with advancing age: 0.3% in the first and second decade, 0.4% in the third decade, 2.7% in the fourth decade, 10.1% in the fifth decade, 20.5% in the sixth decade, 43.5% in the seventh decade, and 60.0% over 70 years of age.

In Korea, J.-H. Paik et al. reported the prevalence of MPB in Korean men of all age groups as 14.1% [8]. The prevalence increased steadily with advancing age, but was lower than that in Caucasians: 2.3% in the third decade, 4.0% in the fourth decade, 10.8% in the fifth decade, 24.5% in the sixth decade, 34.3% in the seventh decade, and 46.9% over 70 years.

From these figures, the prevalence of MPB in Chinese and Korean men was similar to but significantly lower than the prevalence in Thailand. The highest

D. Pathomvanich and K. Imagawa (eds.), *Hair Restoration Surgery in Asians*
DOI 10.1007/978-4-431-99659-0_2, © Springer 2010

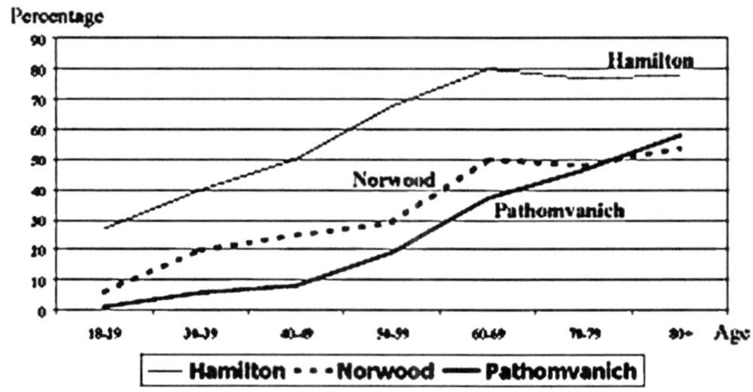

Fig. 1. Comparison of class IV–VII between the Hamilton, Norwood, and Pathomvanich studies. Asians in the Pathomvanich study and Caucasians in the Norwood/Hamilton studies both demonstrated increased prevalence with age. The prevalence of class IV–VII in Asians was lower until after age 80, when it was higher than the Norwood although still lower than the Hamilton groups

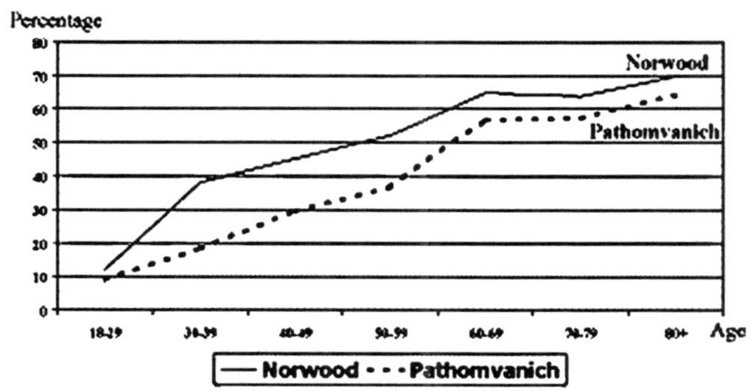

Fig. 2. Comparison of class III–VII between the Norwood study and Pathomvanich study. In comparison to Norwood, the prevalence of III–VII was overall lower in all age groups

prevalence among the Asian groups studied was the 63% in Singapore; this may be attributed to the different nationalities residing in the country or the inclusion of the almost normal Norwood class I in the Singapore study.

In summary, there is a similar increase of prevalence with age among all the Asian groups studied. The majority of Asian MPB also fits into the Norwood classification. The reason for an increase in the prevalence of MPB when compared to Caucasians remains unknown, but change toward a Western diet and lifestyle may play a role. More studies from other Asian countries, such as the Indian subcontinent, Pakistan, and Japan should throw light on the actual occurrence. The wide variation in prevalence rates in the current Asian studies would require a more standardized protocol.

References

1. Norwood OT (1975) Male pattern baldness: classification and incidence. South Med J 68:1359–1365
2. Hamilton JB (1951) Patterned loss of hair in men: type and incidence. Ann N Y Acad Sci 53:708–728
3. Takashima M, Iju K, Sudo M (1981) Alopecia androgenica: its incidence in Japanese and associated conditions. In: Orfanos CE, Montagna W, Stutgen G (eds) Hair research status and future aspects. Springer-Verlag, Berlin, pp 287–293
4. Kakizo K (1969) Correlation between cancer of the stomach and alopecia. Kurume Med J 32:1540–1565
5. Tang PH, Chia HP, Cheong LL, et al (2000) A community study of male androgenetic alopecia in Bishan, Singapore. Singap Med J 41:202–205
6. Pathomvanich D, Pongratananukul S, Thienthaworn P, et al (2002) A random study of Asian male androgenetic alopecia in Bangkok, Thailand. Dermatol Surg 28:804–807
7. Xu F, Sheng YY, Mu ZL, et al (2008) Yang prevalence and types of androgenetic alopecia in Shanghai, China: a community-based study. Br J Dermatol 160:629–632
8. Paik JH, Yoon JB, Sim WY, et al (2001) The prevalence and types of androgenetic alopecia in Korean men and women. Br J Dermatol 145:95–99

Knowing the Difference in Restoring the Asian Look

K. Imagawa

Shoguns, the leaders of the samurai, governed Japan until the overthrow of the Tokugawa Shogunate in 1867. During their ruling periods, hairstyling was used to indicate the social rank and class of Japanese men. There was no obvious male pattern baldness at that time because every man appeared bald as a result of a custom called *sakayaki*. During the coming-of-age ceremony, the potential bald area would be shaved (Fig. 1), and this hairstyle maintained throughout life.

Although it is said that *sakayaki* would help to prevent the buildup of dampness on the head while wearing a military helmet, this style was also popular in classes other than the warrior class. Just like people of our generation, ancient Japanese men might have felt uneasy about becoming bald and found a clever way to conceal the problem. It would therefore be fair to say that baldness was used to imply a positive image of wealth and virtue in Japan. The "pigtail" hairstyle found in the Qing dynasty of China also served to conceal crown baldness. These customs suggest that the onset of pattern baldness was probably unpopular with males throughout the Orient.

Until recently, most believed that the occurrence of male pattern hair loss (MPHL) in Asian people was less than that in Caucasians. Takashima et al. reported that the incidence of MPHL in Japanese is only a quarter of that in Caucasians [1]. Adachi reported 10 years ago that 9.7 million Japanese men experienced MPHL, with a prevalence of 21%. This figure was lower than that in Caucasians (i.e., USA, 34%; England, 36%; Germany, 41%) [2]. According to Inaba, who was well known as an advocate of the sebaceous gland hypothesis, the prevalence of MPHL increased in the Japanese community, probably as a result of the shift to a more Westernized diet. However, no supporting evidence has been provided to substantiate this claim [3]. Pathomvanich conducted a thorough investigation of Thai men and concluded that MPHL in Asians was not as low as previously believed [4] (see the chapter by Pathomvanich in this volume).

It is important to understand the ethnic differences between the scalp and hair of Asians and Caucasians when performing hair transplantation.

D. Pathomvanich and K. Imagawa (eds.), *Hair Restoration Surgery in Asians*
DOI 10.1007/978-4-431-99659-0_3, © Springer 2010

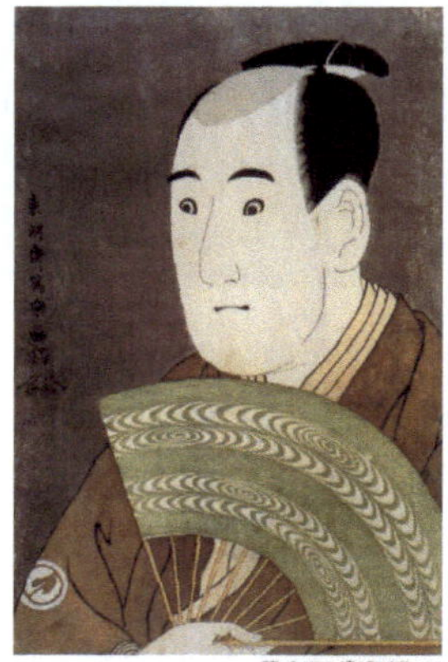

Fig. 1. An Edo period woodblock print: Kabuki actor by Syaraku (1794). The frontal and parietal area is shaved: this is called *sakayaki*

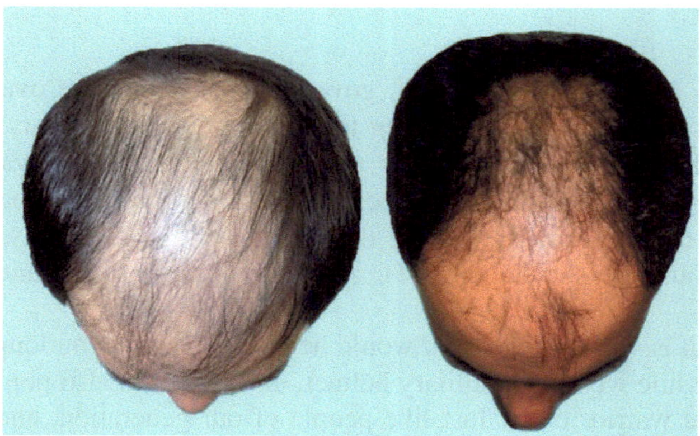

Fig. 2. Comparative anatomy of typical Asian and Caucasian skulls (top view)

Skull and Facial Bone

A typical skull in Asians is short in length but wide in transverse measure. Frontal and occipital projections are less prominent. These characteristics give the Asian skull a round appearance when compared to the more oblong shape of the typical Caucasian skull (Fig. 2).

Although no specific data are available, many hair surgeons would still agree that the average head size of Asian is larger than that of Caucasians [5].

Hairline

The hairline in Asians is different from that of Caucasians because of varied anatomical features, and the following should be considered when creating a natural-looking hairline.

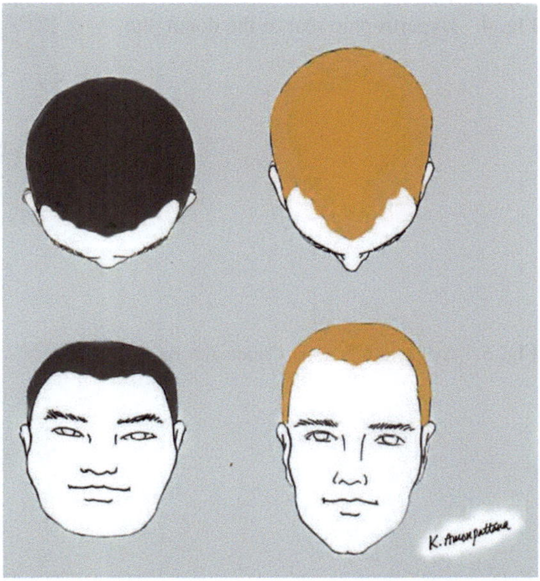

Fig. 3. Difference in hairlines comparing Asians and Caucasians. The typical Asian hairline is flatter than that of a typical Caucasian

1. Basic facial shape: triangular, square, oval, round, and pear shaped
2. Slope of forehead: flat, sloped, curvilinear, and cliff like
3. Frontotemporal angle: wide, acute, and round. The majority of Asians have a wide frontotemporal angle rather than the acute angle seen in Caucasians.
4. Position of hairline: Asian hairlines are, on average, located a little lower than that of Caucasians. The "four fingers rule" in positioning the anteriormost points 8 to 10 cm above the glabella is seldom accepted. As a result, more hair is required in creating the Asian look.
5. Basic shapes of hairline:
   Frontal hairline: straight, U-shape, inverted U-shape, V-shape, and quadrangular.
   Temporal hairline: according to Mayer's classification [6].

The Asian face looks flat because of the round skull, shallow eye sockets, and button nose. These features create a flatter hairline when compared to the bell shape seen in Caucasians (Fig. 3).

Many different shapes of hairline are found in Asia, but the favorite in Japan is the one with a widow's peak called *fujibitai*, referring to the peak of Mt. Fuji [7].

Scalp

According to an old study, Japanese have a thicker scalp than Finnish persons [8]. The overall tough and tight scalp of Asians makes it difficult to apply the blunt dissection technique in donor harvesting. I have given up the use of Haber's scalp

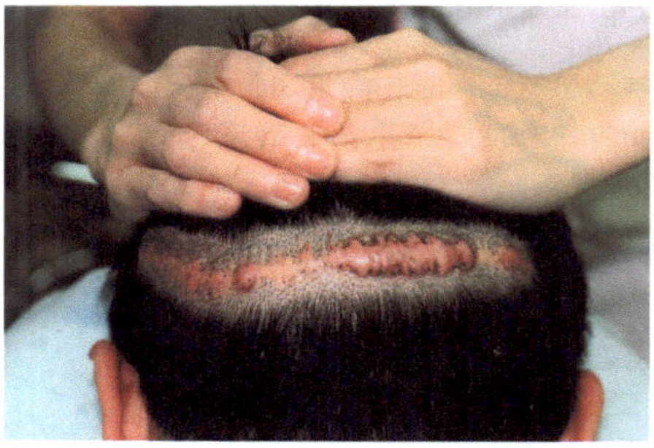

Fig. 4. Hypertrophic scar at the donor site

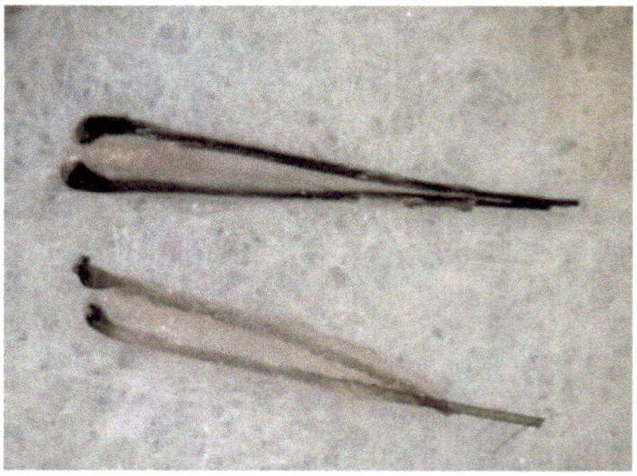

Fig. 5. Asian hair versus Caucasian hair

spreader in Japanese male patients, although this instrument works well in female patients.

In my experience, the Asian scalp suffers a high incidence of hypertrophic scar at the donor site but without any excessive scar formation in the recipient area (Fig. 4). A preoperative test to assess the risk of keloid formation is not required. If a tendency toward keloids is suspected during the initial consultation, aggressive donor harvesting should be avoided and follicular unit extraction (FUE) considered.

Facts About Asian Hair in Hair Transplantation

- The straight hair and fewer number of hairs per square centimeter (Fig. 5) in the majority of Asians makes the scalp more easily visible under direct light exposure. The strong color contrast between the black hair and pale skin also renders it difficult to create an illusion of hair fullness.
- Measurement of donor hair caliber is important in selecting a good candidate. There are several methods for measuring the diameter, but the digital micrometer remains the most practical instrument despite its wide range of readings (Fig. 6). Cole classified hair according to diameter into six groups (Table 1). Asian hair

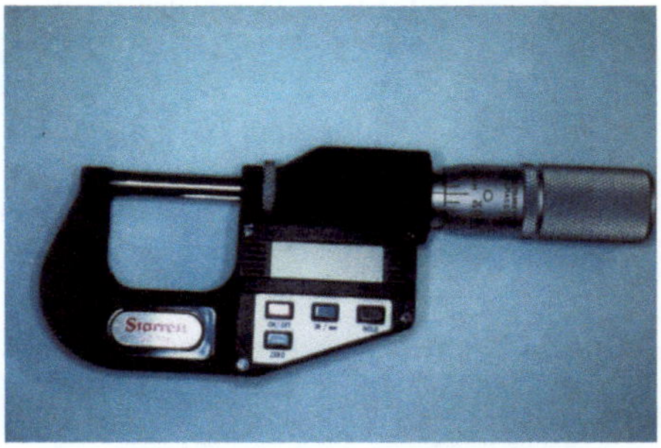

Fig. 6. Digital micrometer

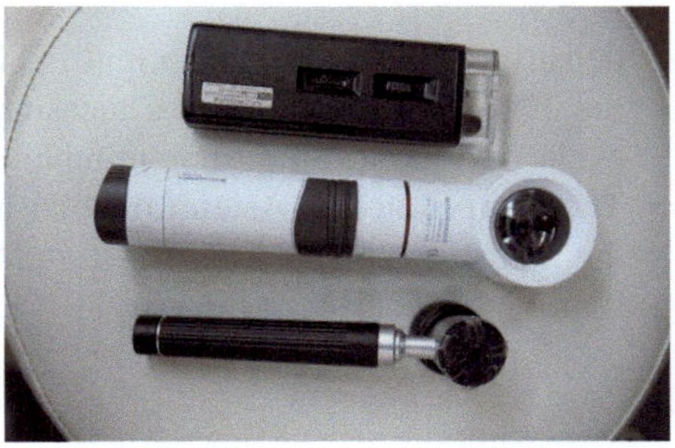

Fig. 7. Various instruments to measure donor density

Table 1 Diameter of hair in micrometers [9]

	Range	Average
Asian	75–78	77
Caucasian	70–75	72

is labeled as "medium-coarse," and the larger caliber contributes to a greater appearance of density. More area can be covered by the same number of follicles. On the other hand, it is more difficult to produce a natural look when multiple follicular unit grafts (MUGs) are transplanted. Even with FUGs, every effort should be made to select the finest hair for the most anterior hairline.

- The distance from the epidermis to the dermal papilla is, on average, 5.0–6.0 mm for Asians and 4.0–5.0 mm for Caucasians. Consequently, the former attract a higher risk of follicular transection during the FUE procedure.
- The donor area hair density must be known to successfully estimate the size of the donor strip. It can be measured by either Rassman's densitometer, dermatoscopy with a 5-mm window, or a video-microscope (Fig. 7). The average donor

Table 2. Donor density in Asians (per cm²)

	Follicular density	Hair density
Mid-occiput	80–90	160–170
Temporal	55–70	100–127

Table 3. Comparison between the characteristics of follicular units (FUs)

	1 hair follicle	2 hair follicle	3 hair follicle	4 hair follicle
Asian	24–30%	50–64%	13–17%	0–2%
Caucasian	14%	52%	29%	6%

density of Asians in midocciput is 80–90 FUs/cm^2 (Table 2); this is lower than the 100 FUs/cm^2 found in Caucasians, and consequently a larger strip must be excised to harvest the same number of grafts.

- The composition of Asian follicular units (FUs) in the donor strips is as follows: the hair: FU ratio in Asians is 1.7–2.0, which is less than that the value of 2.25 found in Caucasians (Table 3) [10–15].

Asian Hair: A Korean Study

J.-C. Kim

1. As most Asian hair is black, coarse, and straight (Fig. 8), hair transplantation is difficult, especially when the skin is light. An Asian with high-caliber hair and a visibly high contrast between hair and skin color requires very small grafts (usually fewer than three hairs per graft) to produce a natural look.
2. Asians have a lower hair density than Caucasians. Korean hairs have a density of approximately 120 hairs/cm^2 in the occipital zone and about 100 at the temple area. Therefore, a larger donor area is required, and available donor hair is limited.
3. Asians have a high proportion of single hairs. The occipital scalp hairs of Koreans consist of 45% of one-hair follicular units, 42% of two-hair follicular units, and 7% of three-hair follicular units. The survival rate of single hair grafts is relatively low compared with two- or three-hair grafts.
4. Because the hair follicles of Asians are longer than those of Caucasians, the probability of transection during donor harvesting and graft preparation is very high in Asians.
5. The hair follicles of Asians are metabolically more active than those of Caucasians. Therefore, the grafts of Asians are more vulnerable to dehydration, preservation temperature, and preservation period.

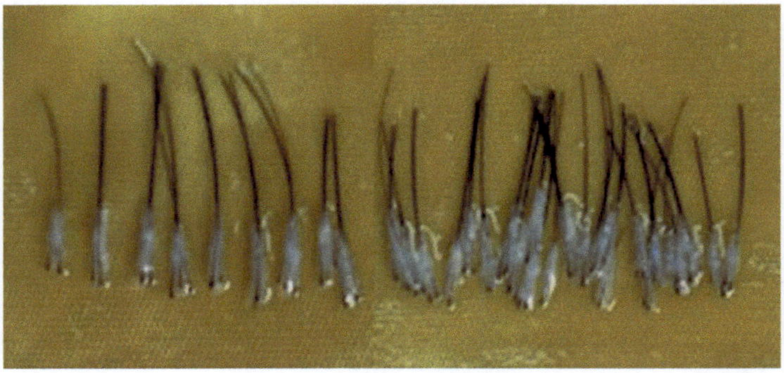

Fig. 8. Asian hair follicles

References

1. Takashima M, Iju K, Sudo M (1981) Alopecia androgenica: its incidence in Japanese and associated conditions. In: Orfanos CE, Montagna W, Stutgen G (eds) Hair research status and future aspects. Springer Verlag, Berlin, pp 287–293
2. Adachi N (1998) Nippon Keizai Shinbun, 28 November (in Japanese)
3. Inaba M, Inaba Y (1996) Androgenetic alopecia. Springer Verlag, Tokyo
4. Pathomvanich D (2002) A random study of Asian male androgenic alopecia in Bangkok, Thailand. Dermatol Surg 28:804–807
5. Leonard RT (2004) Hair transplantation, 4th edn. 6B. Patient expectations and surgical options based on age, ethnicity and sex. Dekker, New York, pp 170–173
6. Mayer ML, Perez-Mera D (2004) Hair transplantation, 4th edn. 15B. Transplantation of temporal points. Dekker, New York, pp 584–591
7. Onizuka T (1971) Surgical hair restoration. In: Plastic & reconstructive surgery series. Kokusei-Do, Tokyo, pp 24–28 (in Japanese)
8. Onizuka T (1971) Surgical hair restoration. In: Plastic & reconstructive surgery series. Kokusei-Do, Tokyo, p 9 (in Japanese)
9. Unger WP, Cole J (2004) Hair transplantation, 4th edn. 10A. The donor area. Dekker, New York, pp 301–337
10. Tsai RY, Lee SH, Chan HL (2002) The distribution of follicular units in the Chinese scalp: implications for reconstruction of natural-appearing hairlines in Orientals. Dermatol Surg 28:499–503
11. Pathomvanich D (2006) Procedures in cosmetic dermatology: hair transplantation. In: Hair transplantation in Asians. Elsevier Saunders, Philadelphia, pp 149–156
12. Imagawa K (2004) Hair transplantation, 4th edn. 15C. Hair transplantation in Asian patients. Dekker, New York, pp 591–595
13. Bernstein RM, Rassman WR (2004) Hair transplantation, 4th edn. 12AA. The rationale for follicular unit transplantation. Dekker, New York, pp 388–408
14. Bernstein RM, Rassman WR (2007) Densitometer and video-microscopy. Hair Transplant Forum Int 17:41–51
15. Wolfram LJ, Dika E, Maibach HI, et al (1997) Ethnic skin and hair: hair anthropology. Informa Healthcare USA, New York, pp 55–77

Part III
Consultation, Planning, and Hairline Design

The Key to Success in Consultation

J. Wong

Surgeons new to the field of hair transplantation, even when well trained and fully competent, may find it difficult to establish a full-time hair transplant practice. Competition is great in North America where there are many established clinics with well-funded and influential advertising budgets. Comparatively, it may still be easier in Asia when the market has not yet been saturated.

From personal experience, it usually takes 3 to 4 years to establish a practice that can generate a profitable income. For a new surgeon with limited experience, the only way to generate business is to set a lower price. Even so, the transplant clinic will need to be subsidized by other financial means before a sufficient client volume is built up. Obviously, this will require real commitment over a considerable period of time.

If you are concerned about the sparse number of hair transplant bookings and the last patient's hair is almost grown out before the next case is scheduled, just hang on! If you really enjoy doing hair replacement, then this is probably the greatest and most rewarding job in the world. The biggest hurdle is booking in cases to complete the first 60 to 80 surgeries. Once you have reached this level of experience, you will have established a competent surgical team. Also, you are able to document and show your work to potential clients. So long as your work is consistently excellent, selling surgeries will not be difficult.

For long-term success, the quality of your work needs to be continually upgraded. New technology has to be reviewed and selectively adopted into your surgical methods, and the surgical team should be continually striving to improve their efficiency. It is much easier to market good teamwork and a superior product. Knowing that their doctor is striving to be the best is also good for the morale of one's staff, who in turn will be encouraged to put in their best efforts.

During a consultation we are selling our teamwork. When we are convinced that our team is consistently among the best, it is easy to convey this message to the patients. They can be impressed by photographs showing our procedure and results.

In North America and Europe, the Internet plays an increasingly important role in providing patient information. As a bare minimum, a well-designed website is essential for any clinic. Most countries have hair websites with an active discussion forum. These are excellent means to showcase one's work and can be a valuable source of surgical referrals.

D. Pathomvanich and K. Imagawa (eds.), *Hair Restoration Surgery in Asians*
DOI 10.1007/978-4-431-99659-0_4, © Springer 2010

People coming in for consultations in the early years of your practice often request a meeting with patients who have undergone the procedure and to see your work. Happy patients with good results and who are willing to meet potential clients are a very valuable resource. They are much more effective than the surgeon or the office staff in casting away any doubts harbored by the indecisive clients and to encourage bookings for surgery.

Most men find it difficult to commit to surgery after one consultation, and follow-up contact is therefore extremely important. A staff member who is very good at building relationships with patients should be designated as the contact person. The idea is not to use high-power sales tactics, but rather to maintain contact with potential clients by one or two follow-up phone calls after the consultation and to truthfully answer any concerns the patient may have.

We provide a complimentary service for patients for whom we have prescribed finasteride medical therapy. A photograph is taken at the start of therapy, and then progress is monitored on a yearly basis. Patients really appreciate the added service, and it provides us with a source for cross-referrals.

Lastly, as physicians we need to do what we believe is in the patient's best interest. Let not the desire to book surgeries interfere with our better judgment.

Hair Restoration Surgery in Poor Candidates

K. Imagawa and J. Wong

Apart from the technique, selection of a good candidate is crucial to achieve the optimal result in hair transplantation. Underlying medical problems or diseases may interfere with the procedures, and special precaution should be taken in these patients. Treatment of medical conditions, however, is not discussed in this chapter.

During the consultation, the potentially achievable results should first be determined by evaluating the hair shaft diameter and donor density as well as scalp laxity. It is important to assess whether the patient's expectation is realistic. Discrepancy between expectation and the actual outcome is a common cause of dissatisfaction in both parties. Four groups of patients deserve special attention.

Body Dysmorphic and Obsessive-Compulsive Patients

These patients will never be satisfied with any results in the long term regardless of the quality of the operation [1].

Young Patients

Among all age groups, patients under the age of 25 years are the most difficult to satisfy. Experienced hair surgeons advise that hair transplantation for young patients should be avoided or postponed. These patients have very high and occasionally unreasonable expectations and are likely to be devastated or distressed by future hair loss. Nevertheless, as male pattern hair loss (MPHL) starts from puberty, it is always difficult to keep these patients from seeking surgical remedies (Fig. 1).

The following guidelines should be taken into account when considering hair transplantation in young patients:

- Set the hairline higher than patient's request.
- Avoid placing grafts in vertex.
- Do not create feminine hairlines by rounding up the apexes [2].

D. Pathomvanich and K. Imagawa (eds.), *Hair Restoration Surgery in Asians*
DOI 10.1007/978-4-431-99659-0_5, © Springer 2010

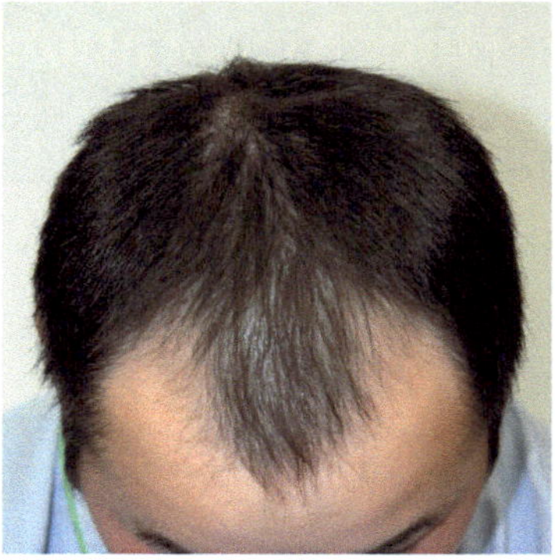

Fig. 1. A 16-year-old man with Norwood class III baldness

On the other hand, recent refinement in surgical techniques when combined with medical treatment may allow a more aggressive approach so long as the patient has good scalp laxity and donor density and is without any family history of advanced MPHL.

Candidates with Very Fine Hair, Very Tight Scalp, and Very Low Donor Density (Fig. 3)

We should resist the temptation to offer the procedure to candidates with very fine hair. The illusion of coverage depends on the diameter of donor hair and the density of grafts transplanted. For the same density, hair 60 μm in diameter can only achieve 70% of the thickness created by hair 70 μm in diameter.

When transplanted with fine hair, older patients with hair loss for years usually appreciate any kind of improvement. On the other hand, patients with high expectations may still complain, "Doc, how come I don't look like the 'After' pictures you posted on your website?" (Figs. 2b, 4b).

One should keep in mind that this group of patients also has the problem of depleted donor reserves for future sessions when hair loss progresses.

Candidates in Norwood Class VI and VII Who Demand Full Coverage

The isolated frontal forelock design is well accepted in Caucasians. Asians in general do not appreciate this hairstyle. They not uncommonly demand full coverage of the bald area even when advised that this would not be possible with the low ratio of donor availability and recipient demand. It is judicious not to perform

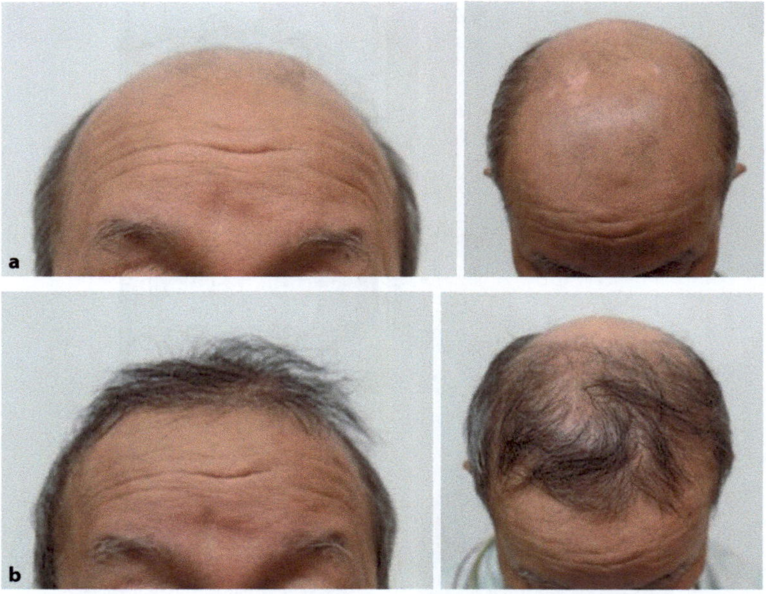

Fig. 2. **a** A 60-year-old man, Norwood class VII: before pictures. **b** At 8 months after one session, 2700 follicular unit grafts (FUGs). The patient's donor hair shaft diameter is less than 60 μm. Although the grafted site still looks very thin, he is satisfied with the result

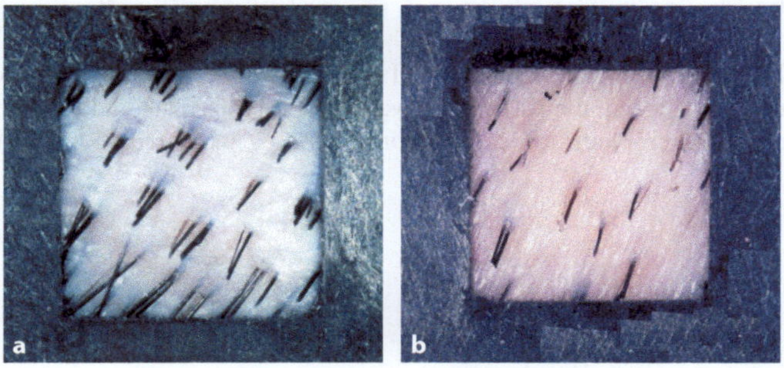

Fig. 3. Follicular units in an Asian: 5 × 5 mm. **a** Good candidate. **b** Poor candidate

full coverage even when the patients insist (Fig. 5). The best option rather is to make a frontal forelock connected to the temporal zones. The worst kind of candidate in this group is the hairpiece wearer. In Asia, the hairpiece is the most popular option for those with baldness. The surgeon should clearly state that "It is not easy to match the huge difference in hair density between hairpiece and hair transplantation."

K. Imagawa

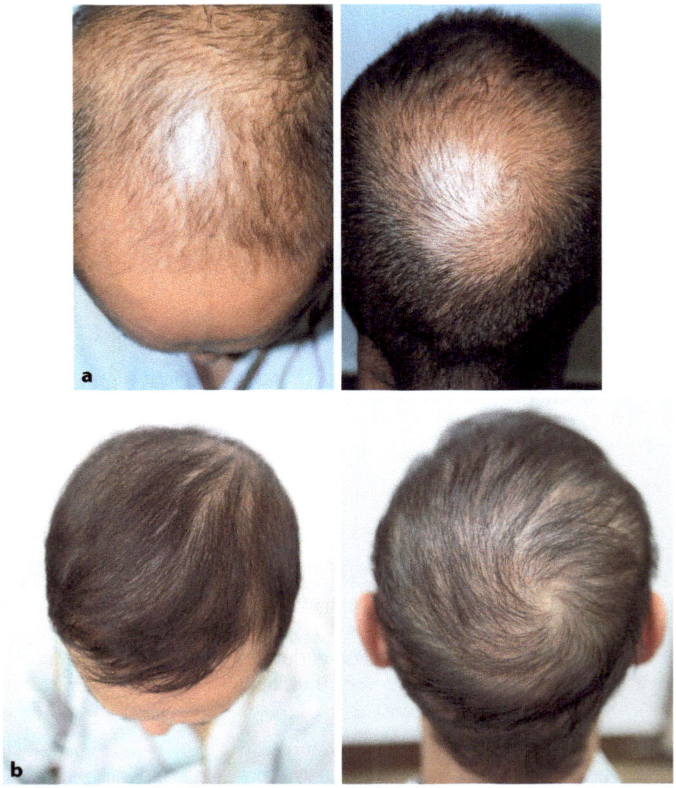

Fig. 4. **a** A 41-year-old man, Norwood class VI: before pictures. **b** After six sessions and a total 8500 FUGs were transplanted, the patient still wants further transplant and refuses medical treatment; he obviously has problems of depleted donor reserves and a wide donor scar

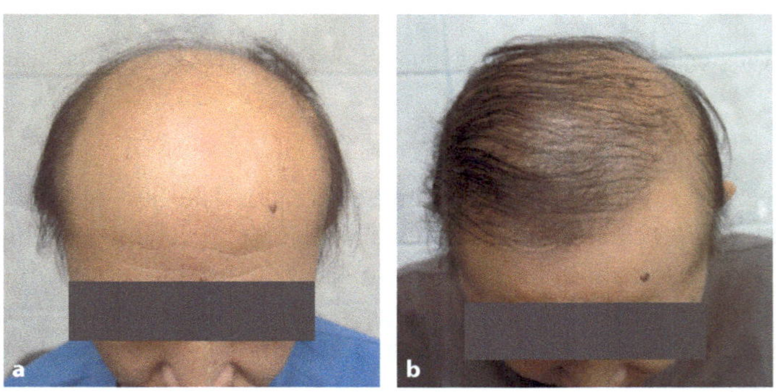

Fig. 5. **a** At 48 years old, class VI. (Courtesy of Dr. Pathomvanich.) **b** At 3 years after hair transplantation: two sessions with a total of 3486 grafts)

We are all aware that unrealistically high expectations will turn even a good candidate into a poor candidate. However, low expectations will not turn a poor candidate into a good candidate. Most Asians with advanced Norwood type VI and certainly Norwood type VII are poor candidates unless their donor density and laxity are such that it is possible to obtain 6500+ grafts over two surgeries. There are very few Asians with sufficient donor density and laxity to do this. It is my personal bias that just putting some hair on top of the head is not enough. There has to be a significant cosmetic improvement from the transplant procedure. Because of its black color and coarse texture, Asian hair needs to be fairly dense to look natural. If there is only sufficient hair for sparse coverage, it will look transplanted even with well-placed grafts.

If we do decide to go ahead with someone we deem a marginal candidate, the person must understand that the hairline needs to be placed high and receded and that only the front hairline and the top will be done during the first surgery. Even with a conservative hairline, it will require 5000 grafts to construct the hairline and provide sufficient coverage to the top area. The grafts need to be packed fairly tightly starting from the front and 300 singles should be saved to soften the back hairline. Even if the patient insists, do not spread the grafts thinly into the crown. Our donor harvest and dissection need to be almost flawless because these people need every single hair for coverage. This requirement means that the team must be experienced and efficient.

Most Asians with advanced hair loss are very difficult and only occasionally will we have someone who can yield 5000+ grafts the first surgery and 2500+ grafts the second surgery. Most of the time, there is insufficient hair to do a decent job.

J. Wong

References

1. Unger WP (2004) The initial interview. 6A. My personal approach to the interview. In: Hair Transplantation, 4th edn. Dekker, New York, pp 166–169
2. Cohen IS (2001) Guidelines for hair transplantation in the young patients. Hair Transplant Forum Int 11:131–133

Preoperative Approach to Preexisting Scalp Lesions

M.J.K.S. Bunagan

Before hair transplantation, a thorough examination of the scalp should be done to assess preexisting scalp lesions that may affect the result of the hair transplantation procedure.

Dermatological diseases that may be present among Asian scalps should be managed before hair transplantation. Among Asians, precancerous and skin cancer lesions rarely develop as compared to Caucasians [1,2]. More common among older Asians (40–70 years) are lesions such as seborrheic keratoses [3,4], which appear as sharply demarcated brown macules or plaques with uneven surfaces over both sun-exposed and covered areas such as the face and scalp (Fig. 1). These lesions can be removed by surgical excision, electrodessication with curettage, or cryotherapy a few days before, or even during, the hair transplantation procedure.

Epidermoid cysts are common cysts that may occur over the head area. These lesions are typically solitary, mobile, skin-colored nodules. Most are slow growing with no symptoms; however, some lesions may become inflamed or secondarily infected. When they are found over the recipient or donor area, recipient slit creation or donor harvesting may cause cyst rupture, leading to a foreign-body reaction [5]. Thus, it would be better to excise the lesion before the hair transplantation procedure.

Lesional growths such as nevomelanocytic nevi may occur over the donor or recipient area. These are benign growths that usually present in darker-skinned individuals as brown or black round or oval lesions with a homogeneous surface and coloration [6]. Small or medium-sized lesions that are not in a visible location need not be removed. Larger lesions in a prominent location, such as a nevus over a patient's hairline, may require surgical excision and wound healing several weeks before the hair transplantation procedure (Fig. 2a). In this particular case, there was a 2-month interval between the excision (Fig. 2b) and hair transplantation surgery (Fig. 2c,d).

Bacterial infections such as folliculitis and furunculosis may occur in skin of color, such as in Asians [7]. These lesions may appear as erythematous papules or pustules over the scalp. Additional exposure to places with high temperatures and humidity may lead to an increasing tendency to develop folliculitis. This condition

D. Pathomvanich and K. Imagawa (eds.), *Hair Restoration Surgery in Asians*
DOI 10.1007/978-4-431-99659-0_6, © Springer 2010

Fig. 1. Seborrheic keratosis over the donor area

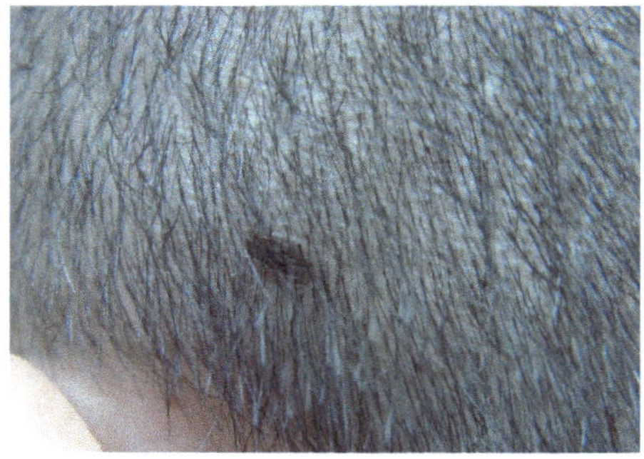

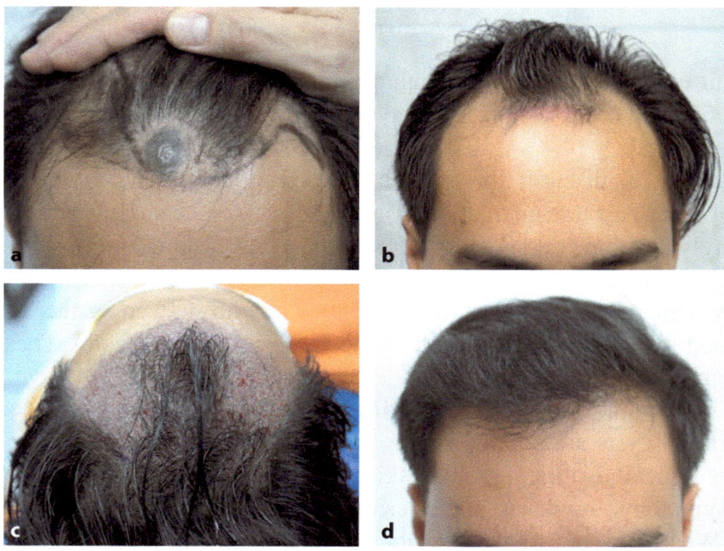

Fig. 2. **a** Intradermal nevus. **b** Nevus excised. **c** After 2106 grafts/3685 hairs. **d** After 9 months

can be treated with oral or topical antibiotics a few days before the surgery. If necessary, the oral antibiotic drug can also be continued during and a few days after the procedure.

Psoriasis is a skin disease also found among Asians [8]. Because the scalp is an area prone to developing psoriatic lesions, care must be taken when contemplating hair transplantation on patients with this condition. If lesions are present on consultation, then treatment is recommended to control the disease before the surgery. The patient should also be advised of the possibility of the "Koebner reaction," a sudden exacerbation of the condition that may develop in the weeks after the surgery. Nusbaum [9] noted that, among several patients with psoriasis for whom he performed hair transplantation, he has not observed psoriatic lesions occurring postoperatively. However, Eisenberg reported this occurrence over the recipient

Fig. 3. Seborrheic dermatitis of scalp

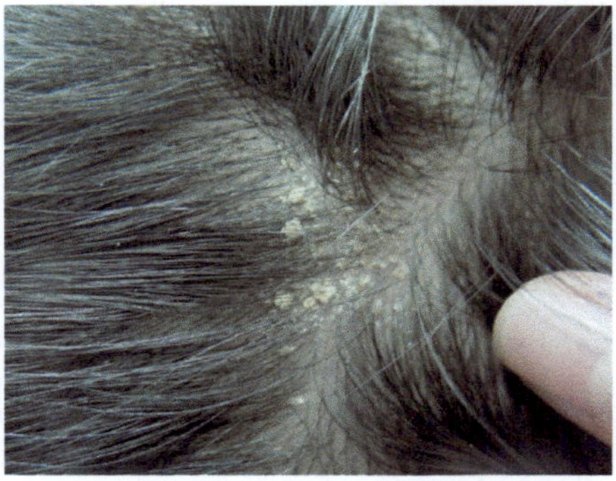

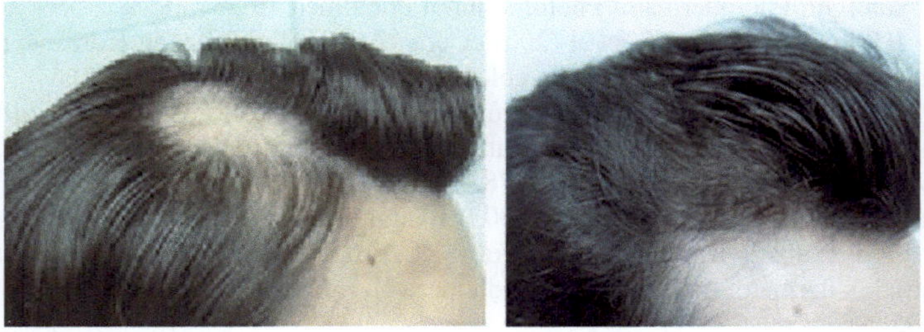

Fig. 4. Inactive alopecia areata before and after transplantation of 722 follicular unit grafts

area in one patient [10]. Shiell, in a personal communication, also reports seeing only one case over the past 40 years among several hundred psoriatic patients, including Asians, so it is not a common complication. No specific studies have been done on the effect of this condition on hair transplantation in Asian patients; however, based on the experience of Pathomvanich and other hair transplant surgeons, there seems to be minimal risk of exacerbation of the psoriasis.

Seborrheic dermatitis is a chronic, recurrent, scalp condition characterized by mild to severe erythema with scaling and pruritus (Fig. 3). One to 2 weeks before surgery, management with the use of tar shampoo and topical glucocorticoids is usually sufficient to control the disease [11].

For cases in which where hair transplantation will be undertaken to restore hair loss caused by an underlying disease, it must be ascertained that the disease process has been stable or inactive for at least 2 years. Transplanting grafts over the recipient area when an underlying disease is still present results in the transplanted hairs being similarly affected. However, once the underlying disease has been resolved or has been stable for a significant period of time, hair transplantation can be performed with a moderately satisfactory outcome. Conditions such as stable cicatricial alopecia may be treated [12,13], or rare cases of chronic inactive alopecia areata recalcitrant to medications. This situation was seen in the case of a patient with alopecia areata of the scalp with a stable lesional condition for 10 years and unresponsive to medical management (Fig. 4). Hair transplantation was done with new hair growth after a few months and without any noted hair loss for the 2 years post operation.

References

1. Byrd-Miles K, Toombs EL, Peck GL (2007) Skin cancer in individuals of African, Asian, Latin-American, and American-Indian descent: differences in incidence, clinical presentation, and survival compared to Caucasians. J Drugs Dermatol 6(1):10
2. Gloster HM Jr, Neal K (2006) Skin cancer in skin of color. J Am Acad Dermatol 55:741–760
3. Kwon OS, Hwang, Bae JH, et al (2003) Seborrheic keratosis in the Korean males: causative role of sunlight. Photodermatol Photoimmunol Photomed 19:73–80
4. Chung JH, Lee SH, Youn CS, et al (2001) Cutaneous photodamage in Koreans: influence of sex, sun exposure, smoking, and skin color. Arch Dermatol 137:1043–1051
5. Silver S, Ho V (2003) Benign epithelial tumors. In: Freedberg IM, Eisen AZ, Wolff K, Austen KF, Goldsmith LA, Katz SI (eds) Fitzpatrick's dermatology in general medicine, vol 1, 6th edn. McGraw Hill, New York, pp 767–783
6. Grichnik JM, Rhodes AR, Solier AJ (2003) Benign hyperplasias and neoplasias of melanocytes. In: Freedberg IM, Eisen AZ, Wolff K, Austen KF, Goldsmith LA, Katz SI (eds) Fitzpatrick's dermatology in general medicine, vol 1, 6th edn. McGraw Hill, New York, pp 881–905
7. Taylor SC (2003) Epidemiology of skin diseases in people of color. Cutis 71:271–275
8. Chua-ty G, Goh CL, Koh SL (1992) Pattern of skin diseases at the National Skin Centre (Singapore) from 1989–1990. Int J Dermatol 31:555–559
9. Nusbaum B (2005) Scalp dermatology for the hair restoration surgeon: dermatologic scalp conditions relevant to hair transplantation. Hair Transplant Forum 15(6):219–220
10. Eisenberg E (2004) Hair loss unrelated to androgenetic alopecia. In: Unger WP, Shapiro RS (eds) Hair transplantation, 4th edn. Dekker, New York, p 78
11. Plewig G, Jansen T (2003) Seborrheic dermatitis. In: Freedberg IM, Eisen AZ, Wolff K, et al (eds) Fitzpatrick's dermatology in internal medicine, 6th edn. McGraw Hill, New York, Chapter 124:1203
12. Imagawa K (2006) Hair transplantation for cicatricial alopecia. J Jpn Soc Aesthetic Plastic Surg 28:122–128.
13. Unger W, Unger R, Wesley C (2008) The surgical treatment of cicatricial alopecia. Dermatol Ther 21:295–311

Planning for Ultra-Refined Follicular Unit Transplantation and the Hairline Design

J. Wong

Although at the time the term "follicular unit transplantation" (FUT) was not yet in common use, FUT, as such, essentially began with Bobby Limmer who introduced graft dissection using stereoscopic microscopes around 1987.

It is impossible to accurately predict the extent and area of future hair loss in every patient. The best we can offer is an educated guess based on family history, the patient's age, and the current extent of hair loss. Those considered poor candidates are usually obvious, but if there are any doubts about whether any particular patient is or is not a suitable surgical candidate, then it is best to delay surgery. Prescribe finasteride and follow them for at least 12 to 18 months to see how well they respond to medical therapy.

How large an area we can cover and the density achievable is dependent entirely on the available donor hair supply. Available donor supply is, again, dependent on donor density and scalp laxity. For example, in patients with good to excellent density and a loose scalp, where it is possible to harvest 4500+ grafts from the first surgery, there is a very good chance that during the course of two procedures we will have moved roughly 6000+ grafts and that this will provide fairly good coverage for most patients with Norwood class VI baldness. Patients with average density and tight scalps are always worrisome because in these individuals we may not get more than 3500 grafts in total over two surgeries. These patients may not be good candidates unless the recipient area is smaller and the patient is unlikely to have extensive hair loss in the future.

The key words in ultra-refined follicular unit transplantation are precision and attention to detail because, regardless of the technique employed, sloppy work will always produce substandard results. In this text, I outline, step by step, the routines that we use at our clinic and the thought processes behind some of the things we do. There are very few references in these chapters as most of the materials presented here have been developed by and are based on the work done at Hasson and Wong.

In this chapter, we start by discussing hairline design. I label hairlines using the distance from the mid-brow to the center of the hairline, and most of our hairlines range from 6.5 to 8 cm. A 7-cm hairline works well in the majority of patients, and

D. Pathomvanich and K. Imagawa (eds.), *Hair Restoration Surgery in Asians*
DOI 10.1007/978-4-431-99659-0_7, © Springer 2010

this is where most of my hairlines are placed. Younger males will often push for a lower hairline. A lower (6.5-cm) hairline may be used if these conditions are met:

1. The current hair loss is not extensive (Norwood class III at most).
2. There is excellent donor hair and laxity.
3. There is no family history of extensive hair loss.

Anything lower than 6.5 cm is too low because people with hairlines this low usually have minimal hair loss and multiple passes may be required to build up sufficient density to recreate a hairline this low. Strong temple points are required to balance a low hairline and, as hair loss continues, further transplants are required, not only for the top but also for the temples. Even if hair supply is not an issue, it is really difficult to make a 6-cm hairline look natural. Because of its coarseness, donor hair looks best at 7 cm or higher. We may place it at 6.5 cm and it may still look alright, but when placed at 6 cm it seems just too coarse and looks out of place.

People with a low (6-cm) residual frontal tuff can be a challenge. With very few exceptions, it is a mistake to design a 6-cm hairline to incorporate the entire tuff. It is far better to design a 7-cm hairline starting behind the tuff. If, after the transplant grows out and the tuft returns and looks a little odd, it can be shaved back or the hair can be removed with a laser. When designing the top hairline we have to remember the hairline consists of the top and temples. The top line has to balance with the temples to achieve a balanced natural look. If the temples are receded and temple work is not indicated because of insufficient donor hair, then a higher hairline, with an upslope, will create balance. A lower, flat hairline will look top heavy (Fig. 1).

The routine I use to draw the hairline is quite simple.

1. Measure and mark a short horizontal line 7 cm above the mid-brow level.
2. Mark a point on this line dividing the face in equal left and right halves. This can be done quickly and easily by holding the marking pen over the nose and bisecting the face into equal halves.
3. From this midpoint draw the top hairline laterally, keeping it on a horizontal plane or a slight upslope when viewed from the front.

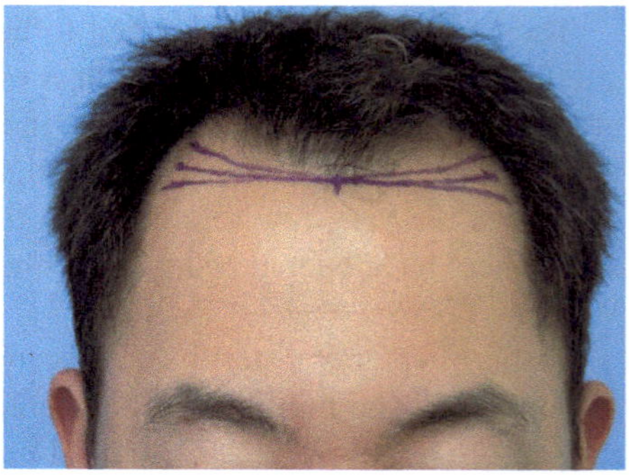

Fig. 1. Patient showing marking for upslope, flat, and downslope hairline design

4. Check from the front to make sure both sides are even and then from the side to see if the line you have drawn balances the existing temples. With practice your eyes will tell you if the top line you chose will balance the existing temples. If the top line looks low when viewed from the sides, you will have to move the top lines up slightly and redraw the top line with a slight upslope.

As a rule, any hairline lower than 7 cm requires strong temple points for balance. If unsure, it is always best to start with a slightly higher design for it is easy to lower a higher hairline but extremely difficult to raise a hairline that was placed too low. Generally, in patients with mild hair loss and average or better donor hair, placing the top line at 7 to 8 cm is safe. If the patient does not object, I generally like to design in a small amount of upslope, thus making it easier to tie the top hairline to the temples without having to extend too far into the temple area. Most Asians will want a flatter hairline however, which is fine but they need to be aware that a flat hairline will only look good with adequate density and that two procedures may be required to achieve adequate density. Patients will often push for a downsloping (juvenile) hairline, and they can be very persistent. Downslopes are seen in African-Americans but seldom in Asians. On an adult Asian this design looks odd, is difficult to correct, and is best avoided.

Because of their black, coarse hair, Asians require more single-hair units to create a natural-looking hairline. I personally prefer to place a minimum of 500 singles at the hairline. One of the benefits of mega-sessions is the large numbers of single hairs that are available for the hairline.

If you are new and starting out in hair transplantation, always keep the hairline high at 8 to 9 cm with an upslope because these early patients who are nice enough to have you practice on their head will need to come back and have their hairlines refined as you (and your team) improve your skill over the next few years. Once again, young people will often insist on a much lower (even 6-cm) hairline that will be a problem after future hair loss. The temptation is to give in and do as the patient wishes. Future hair loss may create headaches for both the patients and yourself as you will be faced with an odd-looking design that may not be fixable and the patient will need a hairpiece to cover up work with your signature on it. To a lesser extent, the same thing could happen even with a more conservative hairline set at 7 to 7.5 cm if the patient should lose hair down to a Norwood class VII pattern.

Laser-Assisted Rapid Hairline Placement

B. Ng

Hairline placement is important. The hairline frames the face and has the most impact on a patient's appearance. Instead of a monotonous universal bell shape, the hairline should be designed to match the individual facial contour for the best aesthetic result.

One of the criteria for a properly placed hairline is symmetry. Differences in symmetry and height from one side to the other impair facial attractiveness [1,2].

Hairline placement can be very time consuming. The patient sees the hairline only after it is drawn. When the design is not accepted the surgeon has to rub off the marking and repeat the whole process. Regardless of the time spent during the consultation, it is difficult to record the exact hairline design on drawings or photographs. The entire procedure has to be repeated again on the day of the surgery.

Use of Landmarks in Hairline Placement [3,4]

Facial landmarks commonly used to assist frontal hairline placement include the following.

1. A symmetrical curve drawn to connect the midfrontal point (MFP) and frontotemporal apexes will outline the hairline [5].
2. Intersection of the nasal tip–pupil line and the MFP–tip of earlobe line marks the temporal point, from which the superior and inferior temporal hairlines are created [6,7].

In real practice, it is difficult to use two landmarks in defining a three-dimensional curve. A flexible tape measure helps but cannot be totally trusted to reach the exact measurement on both sides [3]. Any slight deviation results in asymmetry. Better tools are therefore needed.

D. Pathomvanich and K. Imagawa (eds.), *Hair Restoration Surgery in Asians*
DOI 10.1007/978-4-431-99659-0_8, © Springer 2010

Laser Devices for Hairline Placement

A laser level provides a perfect solution, and two models have been reported in use.

Tripod-Mounted Laser Level

In 2007, Shiao reported the use of a professional-grade laser level mounted on a tripod [8]. The projected horizontal plane of light can "turn corners" and follow the contour of the forehead. A perfectly symmetrical hairline is created instaneously. However, a large room is needed to place the device at the correct distance from the patient.

2. Handheld Laser Device

The device designed by Pathomvanich and Ng has been in use in their clinic since early 2008 [9]. The latest refined model consists of a class IIIA cross-beam laser module (3 V, maximum power 5 mW, 650-nm wavelength) and a batteries box mounted on one end of a 6-in. supporting frame (Fig. 1). The other end of the frame is shaped like a headband and rests firmly on the patient's forehead. By changing the angle of beam projection and its position along the midline, different shapes of hairlines can be created.

Laser-Assisted Hairline Placement: Step by Step

Placing a Feminine Frontal Hairline

The feminine frontal hairline is characterized by an inverted "U" as opposed to the horizontal or upward "U" in the male pattern. The patient is seated in front of a

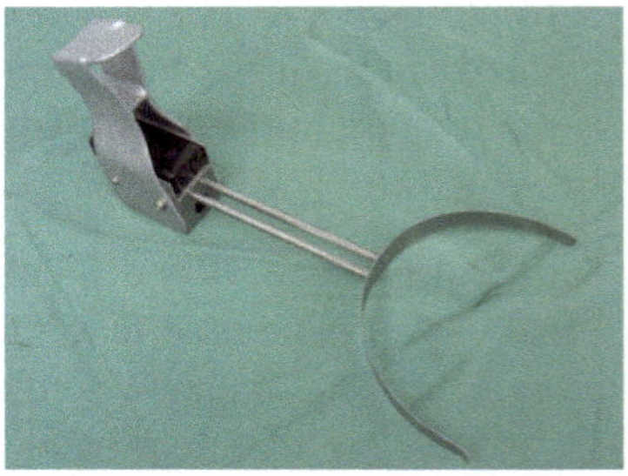

Fig. 1. Latest model of a handheld laser device

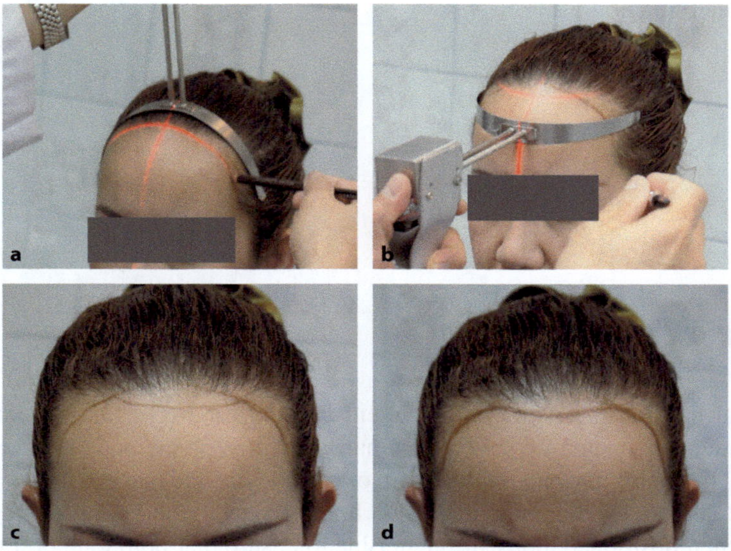

Fig. 2. Drawing a female hairline. **a** Step 1: Casting a downward beam to create an inverted "U." **b** Step 2: Casting a horizontal beam to create another "U." **c** Two curves can be seen. **d** The two lines are smoothed to form a symmetrical hairline

mirror, and a centerline is first defined by aligning the vertical beam with the glabella, nasal tip, and philtrum. Along this centerline the patient marks the lowest point of the desired hairline as the midfrontal point (MFP). The device is then positioned on the frontal region behind the MFP to cast a downward beam (Fig. 2a). The center of the beam must be aligned with the MFP to flow its lateral extensions into the anterior border of the sideburns. Different shapes of hairline can be created by moving the device along the centerline, tilting it forward or backward (Fig. 2b). Symmetry is checked from different angles. The selected curve is then traced and fine-tuned by adding macroirregularities, microirregularities [3], molds, or "V" entrances [6] (Fig. 2c,d).

Placing a Male Frontal Hairline

The centerline and MFP are first located in the same manner. The device is then positioned on the forehead but below the MFP to cast a horizontal or upward beam [3] (Fig. 3). After defining the hairline, the lateral extensions can be connected to the temporoparietal fringes in two different ways: (1) with or without flare, or (2) as a frontal forelock.

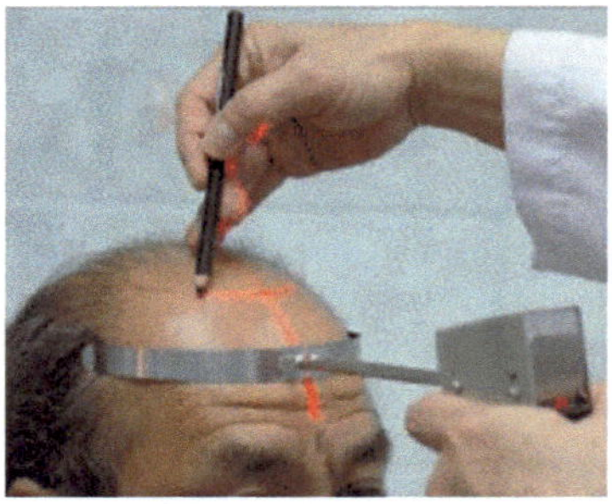

Fig. 3. Drawing a male hairline

Placing a Temporal Hairline

Temporal hairline reconstruction is often required for Mayer class P and R and those patients demanding a low frontal hairline [5]. With the patient's eyes closed, the nasal tip–pupil line and the MFP–tip of earlobe line are marked on the temporal with the laser. Intersection of these two lines locates the temporal point [10].The laser is then positioned along the centerline to ensure that both temporal points lie along its horizontal beam with equal distance from the centerline. The superior temporal hairline is then drawn parallel to the nasal bridge and the inferior temporal hairline parallel to the lateral eyebrow [6].

Placing Eyebrows and Moustache

The uppermost points of the eyebrows are marked on the supraorbital ridges. The device is then positioned along the centerline to cast a downward beam. The symmetrical lateral extensions trace the outer curvatures of the eyebrows. The moustache can be created in a similar way.

Placing a Symmetrical "Scar" in the Donor Site

Even though a strip scar cannot be avoided, some patients prefer to have a symmetrical one when wearing very short hair; this can easily be achieved by using the laser device to outline the incision.

Advantages of Using a Handheld Laser Device

1. Time saving: The patient then looks into the mirror to choose a design before the hairline is traced with a marker. A symmetrical hairline can be completed in less than a minute.

2. Individual design: The hairline described is unique and best suited to the individual's facial contour.
3. Portable: The flat design makes it easy to carry the device in a briefcase.
4. Protective eyeshield is not required so long as the laser is only turned on when in position.

Limitations of the Device

1. The beam loses sight among hair and is thus unable to outline a hairline on areas with existing hair.
2. Symmetry cannot be ensured when the patient's forehead is not symmetrical. In such case one should ignore the vertical aligning beam and adjust the horizontal beam to define a hairline that appears symmetrical.
3. At times an asymmetrical hairline can be more natural looking.The device only serves as a tool, and the surgeon's artistic judgment is still the most crucial in the design and placement of hairlines.

Amendment: Safety Precautions in Using a Class 3A Laser Pointer [11]

Class 3A has a power output less than 5 mW and can damage the eye in less time than the blink reflex. Thus, safety precautions must be taken with its use.

1. Only purchase pointers for which the output power, laser hazard classification, and a warning about potential eye hazard are shown on a label or included in the instructions for use.
2. Never look directly into the laser beam.
3. Never aim the pointer at people or at reflective surfaces such as a mirror. The assistant should not stand behind the patient in case of accidental exposure.
4. The patient should wear a protective eyeshield or glasses if the patient cannot be trusted to close the eyes when facing a laser beam.

References

1. Rose P (2002) Hairline design. Hair Forum 12(5)
2. Springer IN, Wannicke B, Warnke PH, et al (2007) Facial attractiveness. Visual impact of symmetry increases significantly towards the midline. Annu Plastic Surg 592:156–161
3. Rose P, Parsley W (2006) Science of hairline design. In: Haber & Stough hair transplantation. Elsevier Saunders, Philadelphia, pp 55–71

4. Simmons C (2004) Five old lines and three new lines that can help when designing a male temporal hairline or when transplanting the frontotemporal apex. Hair Forum 14(6)
5. Norwood OT, Taylor BJ (1991) Hairline design and placement. J Dermatol Surg Oncol 17:510–518
6. Mayer M, Perez-Meza D (2003) Temporal points: classification and surgical techniques for aesthetic results. ESHRS J 3:6–7
7. Basto F, Graças R (2005) Irregular and sinuous anterior hairline: prior technique refinement and male and female trace parameters. Hair Forum 15(1)
8. Tseng-Kuo Shiao, I-Sen Shiao (2007) Laser-guided hairline design and donor strip marking. Hair Forum 17(2):53–54
9. Ng B, Pathomvanich D (2008) Laser-assisted hairline placement. Hair Transplant Forum Int 18:169–173
10. Brandy DA (2002) A method for evaluating and treating the temporal peak region in patients with male pattern baldness. Dermatol Surg 28:394–400
11. Statement on the use of laser pointers: source of information (2008) University of Toronto, Environmental Health and Safety http://www.ehs.utoronto.ca/services/laserpg/laserptr.htm

When to Restore the Temple Area

J. Wong

The hairline consists of both the frontal and temple hairline, and the best cosmetic effect occurs when one balances the other. In patients with extensive hair loss, that is, Norwood class VI, it is best to design a higher frontal hairline that matches the existing temples because most Asians do not have sufficient donor hair to provide cosmetic density for a low frontal hairline and the temple work is needed to balance a lower hairline.

For these individuals, usually an 8-cm hairline with a slight upslope will blend nicely with receding temples. For individuals with hair loss limited to the frontal area and unlikely to lose the top or vertex, and if the donor supply allows, we may design a flat 7-cm hairline and build up the temples to match. Even with an experienced team temples are difficult to transplant; therefore, if your team has not done much temple work, start with small numbers, perhaps 50 grafts per side, until the technicians gain more experience. Full temple buildups certainly carry the most cosmetic impact, but even partial temple work can look very good, and more can be done later. For the majority of patients, even if the temples are badly faded very fine hairs outlining the original temples can usually be seen using magnification. Most of the time there is no need to design new temples: we simply follow the existing outline.

The majority of people lose more hair on the right temple than the left and often it is only the right side that requires work. There are also slight differences in hair direction in that the hair on the right temple points more posteriorly than that on the left. However, Shiell found the opposite occurrence in his practice in Australia, with more recession on the left side than on the right, and thought it might be related to the way of parting the hair! Further study is needed. Temple hair exits the scalp very acutely; therefore, in areas with no residual hair lay the blade as flat as possible on the skin when cutting to keep the hair's exit angle as acute as possible (Fig. 1).

Temples do not require as much density as the top because the hair lies flat to the skin: a density of 30 to 35 follicular units (FU)/cm may be all that is required. Because of the hair's dark color and coarse texture, temple transplants in Asians will be detectable even with a combination of single-hair and two-hair grafts. This effect can be minimized; we use all one-hair FU. The drawback to using all singles

D. Pathomvanich and K. Imagawa (eds.), *Hair Restoration Surgery in Asians*
DOI 10.1007/978-4-431-99659-0_9, © Springer 2010

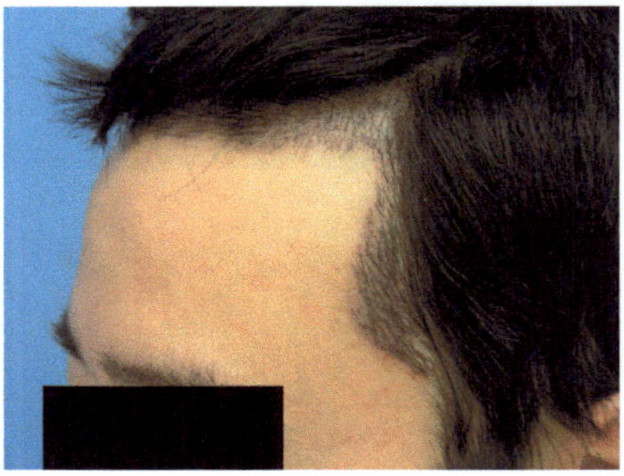

Fig. 1. Temple work: 11 days post operation

is this is much more work and very time consuming, so only small areas can be done. Patients with extensive areas of hair loss at the temples are candidates only if there is a more than adequate donor supply and they are unlikely to have extensive hair loss in the future (traction alopecia). Patients with extensive areas of temple thinning that extend back to the ears are poor candidates because there may be very extensive hair loss in the future and these people have a very limited donor area. If there is any doubt regarding any one individual, it is always best not to do the temple.

Crown: Area of Concern

J. Wong

In a person with extensive hair loss, the first priority is rebuilding the hairline and coverage to the frontal two-thirds of the scalp. As much as some patients may request crown coverage, it is a mistake to spread the grafts out thinner to try and cover the crown because this thinner coverage will produce an obvious transplanted look. After the first transplant, the patient is placed on finasteride and is advised to wait 9 to 12 months to see the growth and density from the transplant. If the patient is happy with the coverage and density with the frontal two-thirds, then if hair supply allows, the crown may be done in the second surgery. The major concern with crown coverage is ongoing hair loss causing a separation between the transplants and the thinning margin. If finasteride showed some regrowth of hair in the crown area, then the patient may be happy to wait and see what finasteride can do in the next 12 to 24 months. For the younger patient, the longer we can delay crown work with the use of finasteride the better. If the crown is transplanted early and should the patient lose down to an advanced Norwood VI or VII, most likely he will not have sufficient hair left to bridge a previously transplanted crown to the receding margin and will be left with an island of transplanted hair. The younger the patient the more difficult it is to predict the degree of future hair loss.

For those who are candidates, they are told that a transplanted crown will always have a thinning look and that only a portion of donor hair can be allocated to the crown. One transplant plus a smaller filler session may be all that can be done, and the remaining donor hair must be saved for future areas of hair loss. Unless their crown loss is very small, Asians seldom have sufficient donor hair for dense crown coverage (Fig. 1).

Nearly all the hair swirls in a clockwise direction, and the swirl is usually off center to the right side. There are usually sufficient fine hairs remaining from the original swirl to show its location and hair flow. If possible, it is easier and better to follow the existing hair direction to replicate the original design. If there are no remaining fine hairs to guide you, then a natural-looking design can easily be done by following the illustrated outline. With the swirl being off center to one side, we have a narrow and a broad side. For the narrow side, the hair arc bends up sharply at the top and points downward (line *a*, Fig. 1); this directional change is rapid. As the hair sweeps downward it changes direction by 90° (line *b*, Fig. 1) and sweeps

D. Pathomvanich and K. Imagawa (eds.), *Hair Restoration Surgery in Asians*
DOI 10.1007/978-4-431-99659-0_10, © Springer 2010

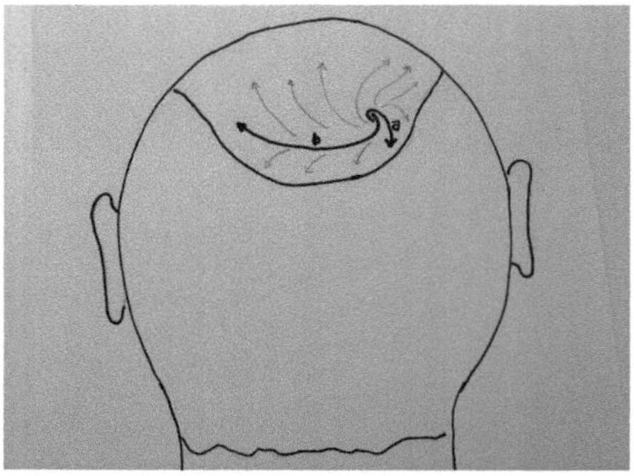

Fig. 1. Diagram of crown swirl. The line shows the direction of hair flow from the swirl

sideways across the broad side before flaring out toward the front and back. At the center of the swirl rapid directional changes occurs within the first 1 to 2 cm, and this area is best transplanted with single follicular units (FUs). Singles give the best density and can accommodate the rapid directional change in such a tight area. Usually 120 to 150 single FUs are used, and these are placed into 0.65- to 0.7-mm slits at a density of 45 to 50 FU/cm^2. Outside of the center, two-hair FUs may be used, and these are usually placed at 28 to 35 FU/cm^2. Larger three- to four-hair FUs are reserved for the outer edges or the downslopes of the crown swirl where the layering effect of the hair can hide and soften the larger grafts.

We label the crown area as upslope, downslope, or sideslope areas depending on the direction of the hair flow. Downslopes are areas where the hair points in a posterior direction and upslopes are areas where the hair points anterior. To plant the downslope and portions of the sideslopes, the patient need to be in the prone position. This may require as much as 2 h, so patient comfort is important. For this we use a padded board with a commercial face ring from a massage table, which works very well.

Should We Use Single or Multiple FU Grafts in Asians?

K. Imagawa

Which will give better results: exclusive follicular unit grafts (FUGs) or a combination of FUGs and multiple follicular unit grafts (MUGs)? So far, no conclusion has been reached in this dispute [1–7].

Advantages of Combining FUGs and MUGs

1. The combination has the advantages of easy donor dissection, shorter operation time, being less labor intensive, and allowing a lower cost per graft for the patient.
2. MUGs are also more resistant to dehydration and rough handling than FUGs as they contain more hair follicles and surrounding supporting tissue [8,9]; this is advantageous in graft survival when the surgical assistants are at different levels of skill and experience.
3. Some surgeons suggest that placing MUGs in the center of the forelock behind the hairline would achieve a better density [4,5].
4. By including more supporting tissue in the MUGs, some claim that this can prevent discarding follicles that are invisible in their telogen phase [6,10].

On the other hand, many hair transplant surgeons believe that FUGs can achieve a much better result. They do not mind paying for the extra labor and equipment, including the microscopes, to prepare the best quality of FUGs. If the ultimate goal of hair transplantation is to achieve a natural look in good density, it would not be an exaggeration to state that such a goal can be completely fulfilled by FUT [11,12].

Disadvantages of Combining FUGs and MUGs in Asians

A few years ago I ceased transplanting double FUs for the Asian patient. My reasons were as follows.

D. Pathomvanich and K. Imagawa (eds.), *Hair Restoration Surgery in Asians*
DOI 10.1007/978-4-431-99659-0_11, © Springer 2010

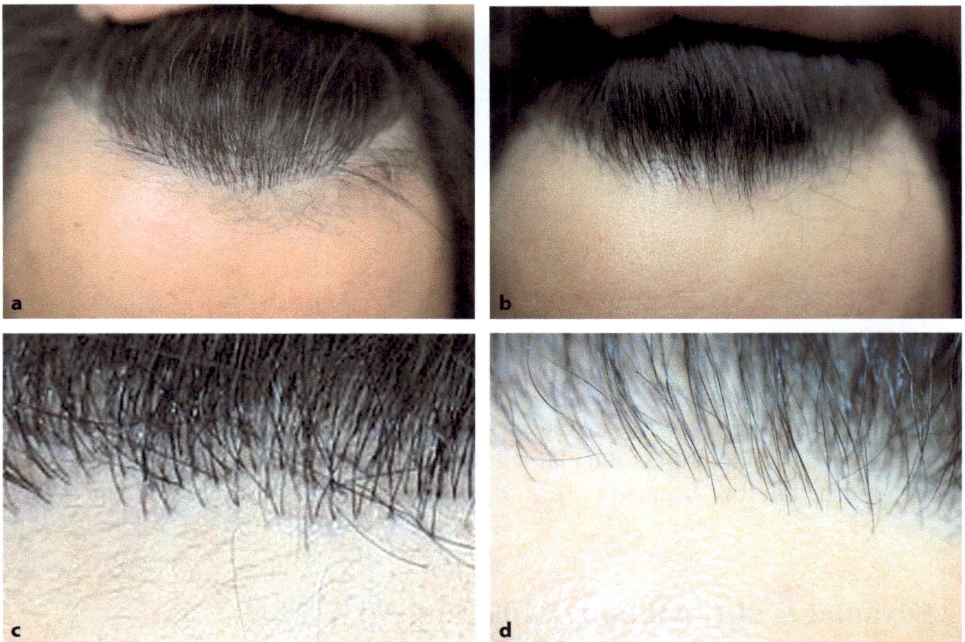

Fig. 1. Comparison between FUGs and Double FUs. **a** Solid and unnatural looking hairline. Hairline was made with a combination of FUGs and double FUs (two sessions). **b** Hairline with exclusive FUGs (one session). **c**, **d** Close-up view of **a** and **b**, respectively.

1. Occasionally, even with FUT, the coarse Asian hair may still stand out as "too thick" for the anterior hairline. Thus, even when using the smallest MUGs, the high skin-to-hair color contrast on the scalp would render it difficult to eliminate any tufting. It is also not easy to use MUGs for restoring the transition zone in women where downy hairs gradually become thicker (Figs. 1).
2. Placing MUGs in the center of the forelock may not always achieve a good density. Asians have a low follicular unit density (FUs/cm^2). As the distance between FUs is greater, the size of a double FU would be considerably larger than that of a Caucasian. Larger grafts require larger slits to house. In return, fewer grafts can be inserted per square centimeter. The average number of hairs per follicular unit is also lower in Asians. When taking all these factors into consideration, it is obvious that the same size of MUG will yield fewer hairs than in a Caucasian. Dense packing with FUGs will achieve a higher density, especially in those with low hair density and low hairs/FU ratio.
3. The larger incisions required for MUGs are more traumatic, and this might increase the intraoperative bleeding and the risks of hyperfibrotic scar formation, as well as "shock loss" in the recipient area [13].

Limmer finds that the statement "telogen hairs are invisible" was not correct. He claimed that these hairs, even at rest, can be seen under microscopic magnification or even with the naked eye when under good lighting. It is therefore unlikely for telogen hairs to be lost in FUT [14].

Conclusions

Although it is the opinion of many Western colleagues that a combination of FUGs and MUGs can give the same results as FUT, I would like to express my personal view that MUGs are of less benefit in Asians in achieving a natural-looking result.

References

1. Beehner ML (2006) The forgotten value of the MFU graft. Hair Transplant Forum Int 16:157–159
2. Limmer BL, Knudsen R, Parsely W, et al (2004) Cyberspace chat... FUT and other techniques. Hair Transplant Forum Int 14:57
3. Elliott VW, Beehner ML, Haber B (2005) Cyberspace chat... Defining multi-unit graft (MUG). Hair Transplant Forum Int 15:213
4. Elliott VW (2005) Grafts containing multiple follicular units have advantages for surgeon and patient. Hair Transplant Forum Int 15:203
5. Shapiro R (2004) Follicular unit transplantation alone or follicular units with multi-FU grafts: why, when and how? In: Hair transplantation, 4th edn. Dekker, New York, pp 435–435
6. Reed WH (2004) Micro-minigrafting: the substance and theory for its use. In: Hair transplantation, 4th edn. Dekker, New York, pp 418–435
7. Rassman WR, Epstein JS, True RH, et al (2008) Controversies: exclusively FU vs. FU and MFU. International Society of Hair Restoration Surgery annual meeting, Montreal, September 2008
8. Gandelman M, Mota AL, Abrahamsohn PA, et al (2000) Light and electron microscopic analysis of controlled injury to follicular unit grafts. Dermatol Surg 26:25–31
9. Beehner ML (2004) Studies of hair survival in grafts of different sizes. In: Hair transplantation, 4th edn. Dekker, New York, pp 261–279
10. Marritt E (1998) The great telogen war. Hair Transplant Forum Int 8:24–27
11. Limmer BL (2005) Transplanted grafts should consist only of naturally occurring follicular unit. Hair Transplant Forum Int 15:203
12. Bernstein RM, Rassman WR (2004) The rationale for follicular unit transplantation. In: Hair transplantation, 4th edn. Dekker, New York, pp 383–388
13. Nakatsui TC (2004) Doing away with incision length. Hair Transplant Forum Int 14:149–150
14. Limmer BL (1997) The telogen hair. Hair Transplant Forum Int 7:12

Advantages of Microvascular Free Scalp Flap Transfer as a Means of Hair Transplantation

K. Ohmori

Hair restoration using a microsurgical free scalp flap was first reported in 1973. Since then, many articles have been written in scientific journals and medical books about this as a method of choice in restoring male pattern baldness and scalp defect [1–16]. Four main types of free scalp flap were reported to meet the different requirements of the recipient site (Fig. 1). The surgical steps are outlined in Fig. 2.

The major advantages of microsurgical free scalp flap are the following:

- Approximately 100 square centimeters of scalp tissue (25 × 4 cm) can be transferred without any conspicuous donor site deformity.
- By careful selection of the recipient site vessels, a normal hair direction can be maintained on the recipient site with normal hair density.
- Because this is a kind of hair-bearing flap surgery, the grafted hair can be appreciated by the patient immediately after the scalp defect is restored.

In other words, as a means of hair transplant, this method can immediately transfer more than 10000 strands of hair in a single operative procedure of around 5 h, and the grafted hair will grow normally with the microvascular anastomosis. In case of hair restoration of the frontal region, the patients can see the results within a week. A much denser result can be achieved compared with the other hair replacement surgeries performed 20 to 30 years ago (Fig. 3).

Despite these advantages, this method has not gained popularity as most hair transplant surgeons were not familiar with the technique. When under the good hand of a skilled microvascular surgeon, this method carries low risk of complications.

One of the reasons that free scalp flap transfer has fallen out of favor is because of the remarkable progress of hair transplantation in the last 20 years. The size of the grafts has been reduced from large punch grafts to mini- or micro-grafts, and then the follicular unit graft. Follicular unit transplantation (FUT) has taken up a central role in the current and future development in hair transplant surgery. The smaller size of the grafts ensures a high-density coverage and a more natural-looking result, especially in restoring the hairline. Its recent significant advancement is described elsewhere in this book.

D. Pathomvanich and K. Imagawa (eds.), *Hair Restoration Surgery in Asians*
DOI 10.1007/978-4-431-99659-0_12, © Springer 2010

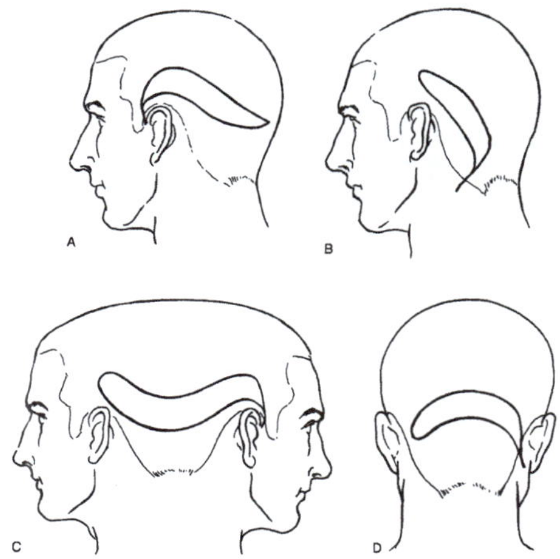

Fig. 1. Four types of free scalp transfers: temporoparietal (**a**); occipitotemporal (**b**); temporo-occipitoparietal (**c**); occipito-occipital (**d**) (From [15], with permission)

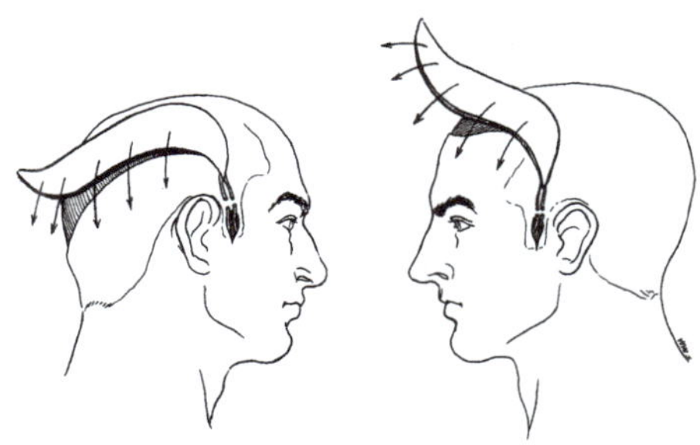

Fig. 2. Free temporoparietal flap transfer is accomplished by microvascular anastomosis. With use of this method, the grafted hair exhibits a normal hair direction. (From [15], with permission)

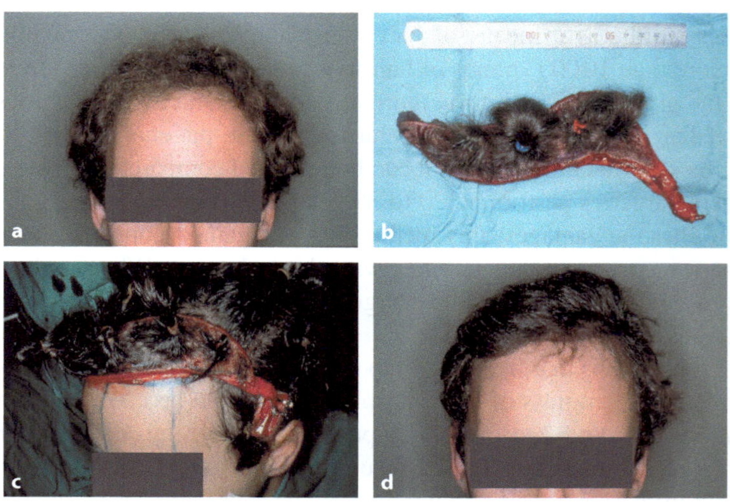

Fig. 3. **a** Preoperative view of the patient with first degree of androgenetic alopecia. **b** View showing free temporoparietal flap. **c** View at the stage of microvascular anastomosis. **d** Postoperative view 1 week after surgery

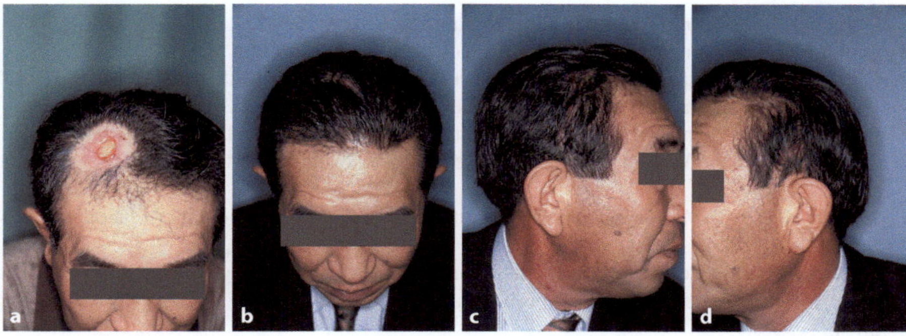

Fig. 4. **a** Scalp defect after unsuccessful treatment of nevus pigmentosus by cryosurgery. **b** View after a left free temporo-occipital flap was transferred. **c** Profile postoperatively. **d** The scar at the donor site is inconspicuous. (From [5], with permission)

Fig. 5. **a** Preoperative view of the patient whose anterior hairline is widely damaged, surrounded by normally dense hair. **b** Postoperative view shows that cicatricial alopecia has been totally covered by a microsurgical free scalp flap

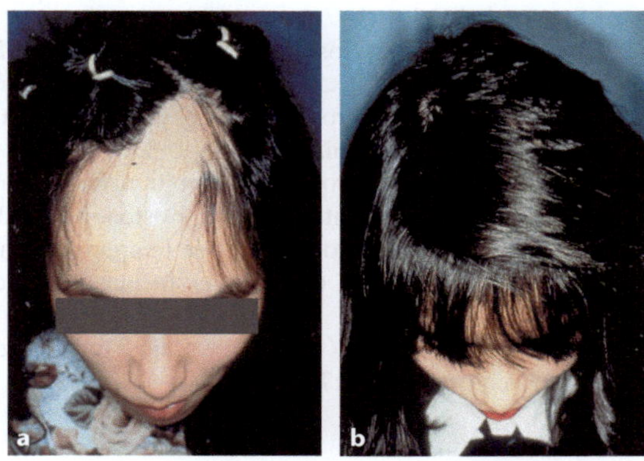

Nevertheless, the microsurgical free scalp flap can still be considered in repairing a scalp defect (Fig. 4). In fact, this can be regarded as the first choice in restoring a severely or widely damaged anterior hairline caused by injuries, especially for women (Fig. 5). Similarly, for patients with limited first-degree androgenetic alopecia, microsurgical free scalp flap may still play a role as more strands of hair can be transferred than in FUT. Moreover, the densely grafted hair from the flap will blend in very well with the surrounding hair. After the flap is created, a few rows of FUT can be added on to achieve a very natural looking anterior hairline.

References

1. Harii K, Ohmori K, Ohmori S (1974) Successful clinical transfer of ten free flaps by microvascular anastomoses. Plast Reconst Surg 53:259–270
2. Harii K, Ohmori K, Ohmori S (1974) Hair transplantation with free scalp flap. Plast Reconst Surg 53:410–413

3. Ohmori K (1980) Free scalp flap surgery. Ann Plast Surg 5:17–23
4. Ohmori K (1980) Free scalp flap. Plast Reconstr Surg 65:42–49
5. Ohmori K (1982) Application of microvascular free flaps to scalp defects. In: Whitaker LA (ed) Clinics in plastic surgery, vol 9. Saunders, Philadelphia, pp 263–268
6. Ohmori K (1983) Hair transplantation with microsurgical free scalp flaps. In: Williams B (ed) Transactions of the VIII international congress of plastic and reconstructive surgery, Canada, p 682
7. Ohmori K (1992) Microsurgical free scalp flaps in surgery for male pattern baldness. Plast Surg 1:581–583
8. Ohmori K (1987) Restoration of the anterior hairline with microsurgical free scalp flaps. In: Stark RB (ed) Plastic surgery of the head and neck. Churchill Livingstone, New York, pp 38–45
9. Ohmori K (1987) Microsurgical scalp reconstruction. In: Brent B (ed) The artistry of reconstructive surgery. Mosby, St. Louis, pp 477–487
10. Unger WP, Nordstrom REA (1988) Microsurgical free scalp flap and androgenic alopecia. In: Hair transplantation, 2nd edn. Dekker, New York, pp 661–674
11. Kobayashi S, Ohmori K (1988) Chronic abscess and partial scalp defect treated by vascularized free omental transfer. In: Brunelli G (ed) Textbook of microsurgery. Masson SpA, Milano, pp 1035–1038
12. Ohmori K (1989) Microsurgical free scalp flaps. In: Baker SR (ed) Microsurgical reconstruction of the head and neck. Churchill Livingstone, New York, pp 269–285
13. Ohmori K (1990) Microvascular free scalp flaps. In: McCarthy JG (ed) Plastic surgery, vol 2. Saunders, Philadelphia, pp 1531–1533
14. Ohmori K (1990) Microvascular free transfer of temporo-occipital scalp flaps. In: Encyclopedia of flaps, vol 1. Little, Brown, Boston, pp 32–36
15. Ohmori K (1991) Microsurgical free temporoparietal flaps in surgery for male pattern baldness. In: Whitaker LA (ed) Clinics in plastic surgery, vol 18. Saunders, Philadelphia, pp 791–796
16. Boo-Ghai K, Zhang, D (1983) Free scalp flap in correcting alopecia of temporofrontal region. Plast Reconstr Surg 71:736

Is There a Place for Scalp Flap in Modern Hair Restoration Surgery?

K. Imagawa

Punch graft has never been popular in Asian countries as its corn-row appearance is more conspicuous with the coarse black hair of Asians. On the other hand, scalp flaps were well accepted and have enjoyed popularity since the 1970s. There are many types of scalp flap (Table 1); however, I will concentrate on my experience with the Fleming and Mayer flap, which is the modification of Juri's flap first described in 1980 [1]. When compared with the punch graft, flaps have the advantages of achieving immediate results, no temporal hair loss, outstanding density, and the possibility to re-allocate a large amount of hair.

However, the rapid innovations of hair transplantation techniques over the past 10 years have eclipsed the predominance of scalp flaps. Mega-sessions and maxi-sessions have arrived on stage and are now routinely available in most hair transplant centers. The once dominant position of the flaps is thereby lost to the latest follicular unit transplantation (FUT) technique, by which a large amount of hair can be transplanted over a large area of baldness and the final result is natural with no recipient scar.

In contrast to earlier times when three or four sessions were required, the current trend in FUT dense packing can achieve good density in just one or two session(s). This change has further eroded another advantage of flaps: super density.

The donor:recipient ratio in scalp flap is 1 : 1, meaning the flap is used to create an area of hair of the same size. The new concept of "appearance of fullness" introduces the idea that illusion of fullness can be achieved even when grafts are replaced at half the donor density. Contemporary hair transplantation has the advantage to cover twice the recipient size compared to using a scalp flap. In other words, a donor:recipient ratio of 1 : 2 is now achievable in hair transplantation. We must keep in mind that male pattern hair loss (MPHL)/female pattern hair loss (FPHL) is always progressive while the donor hair is limited and may be depleted, at least until the time when cloning becomes more practical.

The downfall of scalp flaps also stems from their significant complications and morbidities. The overwhelming criticism on the Internet has discredited the scalp flap. It is regrettable that most of the unsuccessful cases are actually performed by unskilled or inexperienced surgeons.

D. Pathomvanich and K. Imagawa (eds.), *Hair Restoration Surgery in Asians*
DOI 10.1007/978-4-431-99659-0_13, © Springer 2010

Table 1. Various types of hair-bearing flaps

1.	Temporo-parieto-occipital (TPO) flap	Juri 1974
2.	Occipital flap	Juri 1975
3.	Temporo-parietal (TP) flap	Elliott 1977
4.	Microsurgical free flaps	Ohmori 1980
5.	Superior-based temporo-parietal flap and temporal flap	Nataf 1984
6.	Expanded BAT & TAT flaps	Anderson 1987

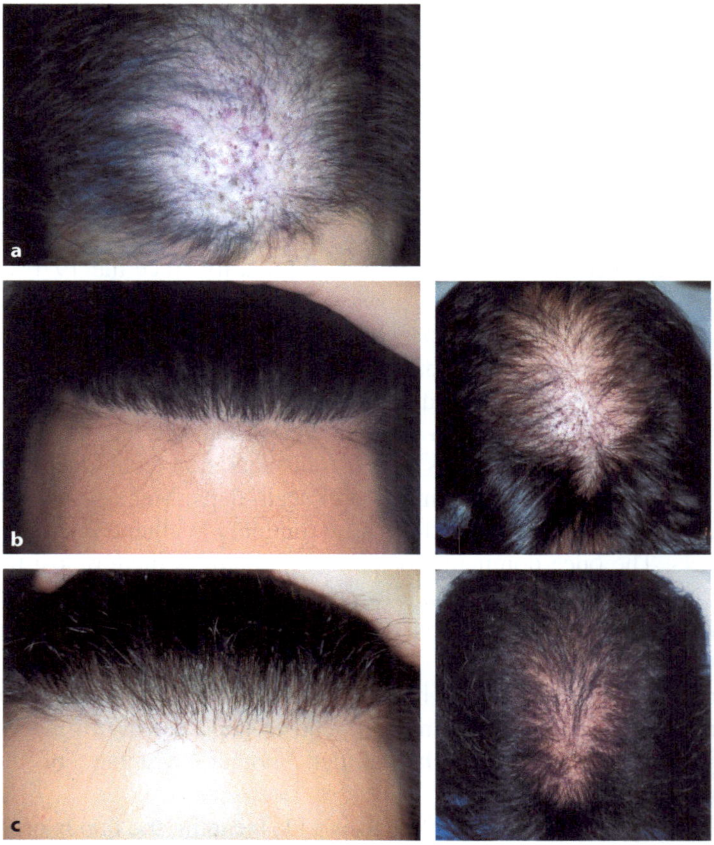

Fig. 1. Temporo-parieto-occipital (TPO) flap. **a** This patient underwent several sessions of artificial fiber implantation, and an inflammatory process was seen. **b** Six months after the rotation of TPO flap (front and top views). **c** These procedures were performed in the late 1990s, and this case was treated by hair transplantation. One session of mini-grafts and micro-grafts (1600) was performed to camouflage the abrupt hairline and alopecia behind the flap

Under these circumstances, the scalp flaps can hardly compete with FUT in treating MPHL. Even, when recommended by the hair surgeons, few patients would accept this type of procedure. All other conditions that were previously treated by scalp flaps, such as congenital defect, trauma, burns, and iatrogenic alopecia, can now be repaired by hair transplantation (Figs. 1a–c, 2a–d).

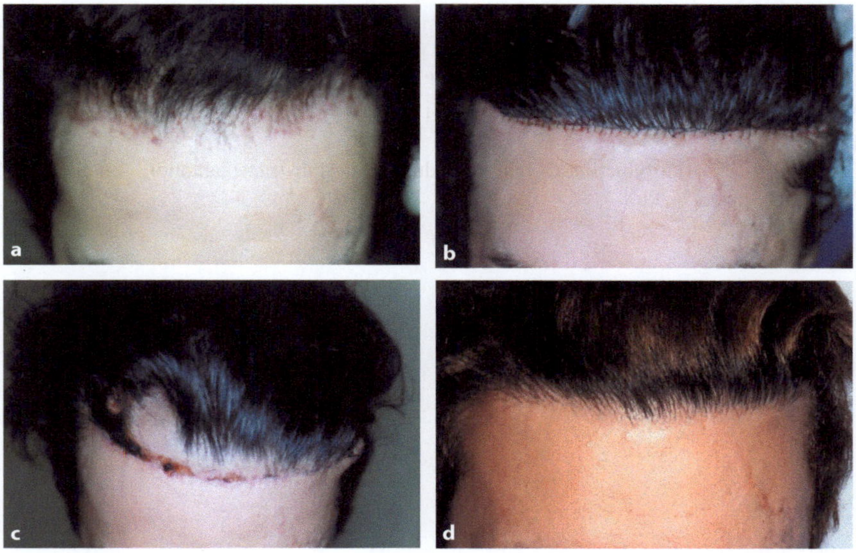

Fig. 2. Temporo-parieto-occipital (TPO) flap. **a** This patient underwent one session of artificial fiber implantation, and an inflammatory process was seen. **b** Immediately after the rotation of TPO flap. **c** Telogen effluvium and partial necrosis of the distal part of the flap was seen. He was a heavy smoker and disregarded our warning of "No smoking." **d** Two years after two sessions of mini- and micro-grafts for the repair. The procedures were performed in the late 1990s, and this case is now treated by hair transplantation

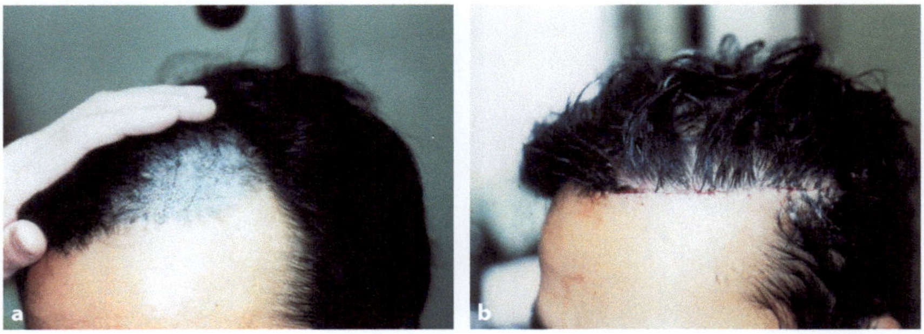

Fig. 3. Left temporo-parietal (TP) flap. **a** This patient had a blue nevus at his left hairline. **b** Immediately after the rotation of the TP flap. The procedure was performed in the early 1990s, and this case still may be an indication for the flap

So is there any other application for the scalp flaps? These can be considered as an alternative procedure for cases where the affected part needs to be excised, such as naevi and tumors (Fig. 3a,b).

I would like to conclude by quoting a statement from Seery: "Yes, there is a place for the scalp flaps but that they should play a small role in the surgical treatment of alopecia seems reasonable" [2].

References

1. Mayer TG, Fleming RW (1992) Aesthetic and reconstructive surgery of the scalp. Mosby Year Book, St. Louis
2. Seery GE (2004) Introduction to flap procedures. In: Hair transplantation, 4th edn. Dekker, New York, pp 795–796

Part IV
Medical Treatment

Medical Treatment of Hair Loss

M.J.K.S. Bunagan

Male Pattern Hair Loss

Currently, there are only two drugs approved by the U.S. Food and Drug Administration (FDA) for the treatment of pattern hair loss in men: oral finasteride and topical minoxidil.

Finasteride

Finasteride inhibits type II 5-alpha-reductase, the enzyme that converts testosterone into dihydrotestosterone (DHT), which is responsible for the progressive miniaturization of hair follicles seen in male pattern hair loss.

Clinical studies have shown that finasteride 1 mg/day slowed hair loss and increased hair growth in men with mild to moderate pattern hair loss [1,2]. Results can be seen in 4 to 6 months. Long-term studies also revealed that the continuous use of finasteride decreases the likelihood of developing further visible hair loss [3,4]. Discontinuation of the drug leads to return to pretreatment condition.

Among Asians a study done on Japanese men with pattern hair loss showed that 1 mg of finasteride taken once daily slowed hair loss and improved hair growth in Japanese men with male pattern hair loss [5]. Finasteride treatment was generally well tolerated among this group. Similar results were seen among Taiwanese men with male pattern hair loss in whom 1 year of continuous intake of finasteride resulted in decrease of the progression of hair loss in the majority of patients and observable hair growth in more than 50% [6].

The only notable side effects in various studies were decreased libido, erectile dysfunction, gynecomastia, and breast tenderness. Small breast nodules have been reported by some patients, but these have proved benign on biopsy. These adverse events were seen only in a very small percentage of patients and were noted to disappear soon after finasteride was stopped [1].

The prostate-specific antigen (PSA) test is highly recommended before starting finasteride in men aged 40 years or older.

D. Pathomvanich and K. Imagawa (eds.), *Hair Restoration Surgery in Asians*
DOI 10.1007/978-4-431-99659-0_14, © Springer 2010

Minoxidil

Topical minoxidil was the first FDA-approved drug for male pattern hair loss. Even after some 20 years, the exact mechanism of action of minoxidil in hair restoration is still unknown.

Various studies have shown the efficacy of topical minoxidil on mild to moderate hair loss. Significant regrowth of terminal and indeterminate hairs and a progressive decrease in vellus hair counts was seen in patients using the 2% and 3% solutions [7,8].

Among Asians, a study involving Chinese patients showed moderate hair growth in 22% and minimal growth in 59%. All patients noted their hair shedding decreased after the regular application of the drug for 1 to 3 months [9].

Currently, 5% topical minoxidil is preferred over 2% to 3% solutions. Clinical trials have shown that minoxidil 5% was clearly superior to 2% topical minoxidil in increasing hair regrowth. In addition, there was also an earlier response to treatment with the 5% solution than with the 2% [10].Topical minoxidil (5% and 2%) was well tolerated by the men in these various trials without evidence of systemic effects [7–10].

Under Investigation

Dutasteride

A clinical trial done on 17 pairs of identical twins showed that dutasteride significantly improved hair growth at 1 year compared to placebo. This finding was based on analysis of the investigator's assessment and patient self-assessment questionnaires [11].

Another study revealed that dutasteride increased target area hair count versus placebo in a dose-dependent fashion and that dutasteride 2.5 mg was superior to finasteride at 12 and 24 weeks. The increase in hair growth was likewise supported by expert panel photographic review and investigator assessment [12].

Dutasteride is currently utilized for the treatment of benign prostatic hypertrophy (BPH) and not yet approved for male pattern hair loss. The commercially available dose is 0.5 mg/capsule with a half-life of approximately 4 to 5 weeks at steady state, which is much longer than the 6- to 8-h half-life of finasteride. In the pattern hair loss study comparing dutasteride and finasteride there was no occurrence of impotence with either medication. Some decrease in libido was seen in 9 of 71 men in the dutasteride 2.5 mg group, whereas this side effect was seen in 3 of 70 patients in the finasteride group. In this study the adverse effect was described as mild to moderate in severity and often resolved with continuation of dutasteride. In the clinical trials of dutasteride for BPH, other possible adverse effects reported were gynecomastia and reduced sperm count. Thus, the benefit of using this drug for MPHL must be weighed against the possible side effects.

Female Pattern Hair Loss

Topical minoxidil is the only FDA-approved drug for female pattern hair loss.

Minoxidil

Currently, only 2% topical minoxidil is FDA approved for the treatment of female pattern hair loss. A clinical study comparing 2% minoxidil lotion with placebo has shown that 2% minoxidil applied twice daily resulted in mild to moderate regrowth in women with pattern hair loss [13]. Possible side effects include contact dermatitis and facial hypertrichosis, seen in a minority of patients. The hypertrichosis completely resolves a few weeks to months after stopping the medication [14].

Among Asian women, the only clinical trial done was on the efficacy of 1% topical minoxidil versus placebo for androgenetic alopecia in Japanese female patients. The results showed a significant increase of non-vellus hair counts in the minoxidil group [15].

A study comparing 2% and 5% topical minoxidil showed that at week 48 there was no statistically significant difference based on the investigator's global assessment; however, the 5% topical minoxidil group demonstrated statistical superiority over the 2% topical minoxidil group in the patient assessment of treatment benefit. In this study, both concentrations of topical minoxidil were well tolerated without evidence of systemic adverse effects [16].

Under Investigation

Antiandrogens

A clinical study on the effect of spironolactone and cyproterone acetate on women with female pattern hair loss showed that 35 (44%) had hair regrowth, 35 (44%) had no clear change in hair density before and after treatment, and 10 (12%) experienced continuing hair loss during the treatment period. For this study, 88% of women receiving oral antiandrogens had no progression of their FPHL [17].

Medical Treatment and Hair Transplantation

The use of minoxidil in conjunction with hair transplantation has been reported as beneficial by 11 international hair transplant surgeons in a round table consensus.

According to the group, minoxidil helps in stabilizing hair loss, increasing the number of hairs in an anagen phase, increasing hair weight and density by enlarging miniaturized suboptimal follicles, making transplanting easier and decreasing post-surgical telogen effluvium. Guidelines for use included discontinuation 3 days before surgery and resumption 1 to 2 weeks after the procedure [18].

In a double-blind clinical trial, 2% minoxidil versus placebo applied before hair transplantation reportedly resulted in less hair shed from transplanted grafts during the postsurgical shedding period [19].

The effect of finasteride on hair transplantation outcome was also studied. In this clinical trial 1 mg of finasteride was continuously taken from 4 weeks before hair transplantation surgery up to 48 weeks postoperation, at which time evaluation of scalp hair was done. Results at 48 weeks showed that there was significant improvement of scalp hair through photographic assessment and hair counts. This study concludes that finasteride improves scalp hair surrounding the hair transplant and increases hair density [20].

Asian Herbal Medications Being Investigated for Hair Loss in Men and Women

Herbal medicines have long been used by Asians for the treatment of various medical conditions including hair loss. Various preliminary studies on animal models have been undertaken to explore the hair growth-promoting effects of some of these herbal medications.

For instance, in India, *Cuscuta reflexa* (Roxb.), *Citrullus colocynthis* (Schrad.), and *Eclipta alba* (Hassk.) are herbs traditionally acclaimed for their hair growth-promoting potential. A study done combining the three herbs showed that on shaved rats the hair growth initiation time was markedly reduced, to one-third, and analysis of the hair growth cycle after treatment exhibited a greater number of hair follicles in anagenic phase compared with control, thus showing some potential for the possible treatment of hair loss [21].

Another study evaluated the petroleum ether extract of leaves and flowers of *Hibiscus rosa-sinensis* for its potential on hair growth by in vivo and in vitro methods. Results showed that the leaf extract had more hair growth potency than the flower extract [22].

Eclipta alba Hassk is a well-known Ayurvedic herb with purported claims of hair growth promotion. The extract of this herb and minoxidil 2% solution for comparison were applied on the shaved denuded skin of albino rats. Results showed that hair growth initiation time was significantly reduced, to half, on treatment with the extracts, and quantitative analysis of hair growth exhibited a greater number of hair follicles in anagenic phase as compared to minoxidil [23].

A study by Rho et al. examined the effects of 45 plant extracts traditionally utilized in Oriental medicine to treat hair loss. Results showed that, among the tested plant extracts, *Asiasari radix* showed the most potent hair growth stimulation in mice experiments. According to this study, this hair growth effect may result from its regulatory effects on both cell growth and growth factor gene expression [24].

In South Korea, a research study screened natural plant extracts having inhibitory activities of 5-alpha-reductase type 2 and demonstrated their biological function in androgen-related animal models. *Thujae occidentalis* semen (TOS) extract demonstrated inhibitory activity for 5-alpha-reductase type 2, suggesting that TOS extract could be used as an effective agent for male pattern baldness [25].

A study on green tea with its major constituent of epigallocatechin-3-gallate (EGCG) showed that it promoted hair growth in hair follicles ex vivo culture and the proliferation of cultured human dermal papilla cells, resulting in human hair growth [26].

A popular Chinese hair product containing Aralia Quinquefolia, Astragalus Glycyphyllos, Angelica Archangelica Root, Zingiber Officinale, Carya Alba, Rhizome of Szechwan Lovage, Corthamis Tinctorius, Paorulca Glandulosa, and Salvia Officinalis has long been used for the treatment of hair loss. Results in one published study showed that in normal rats, guinea pigs, and rabbits, the weight of regrown hairs in the shaved areas of this product's treatment group was significantly heavier than the comparison alcohol group [27]. Other laboratory data on other hair growth parameters are lacking. Reported clinical trials have been done in several Chinese hospitals; however, full, published papers of these studies are not readily available.

These herbal medications show potential in promoting hair growth; however, further studies must be done to verify their effectiveness in the treatment of hair loss.

Conclusion

For most men and women with pattern hair loss, the use of medications may improve their present condition and halt or at least delay this ongoing process.

Currently based on research studies, the use of finasteride 1 mg orally in conjunction with 5% topical minoxidil is recommended for male pattern hair loss. For female pattern hair loss, the use of topical minoxidil 2% or 5% twice daily would be beneficial. These drugs are especially efficacious in patients with mild to moderate hair loss where the areas affected by thinning may experience an increase in hair counts, improvement in hair caliber, or at the very least, prevention of further shedding of existing hair. In addition, the use of these drugs in conjunction with hair transplantation seems to be advantageous. For scalp areas devoid of hair, the main treatment option would be hair transplantation, while the aforementioned medications would mostly improve the existing hair surrounding the transplanted hairs.

The Use of Herbal Medicine

J.-C. Kim

There are also a number of non-FDA-approved treatments currently available that supposedly improve circulation and nutrition in the scalp. These therapies are sold over the counter or via the Internet as treatment for male pattern baldness, but do not have efficacy proven by scientific study.

Many herbal products sold to treat male pattern baldness make the claim of affecting DHT levels. Herbal products usually contain much phytoestrogen, flavonoids, and polyunsaturated fatty acids, which can inhibit the production of DHT. However, there are no scientific studies showing effectiveness of herbal products in treating male pattern baldness.

References

1. Kaufman KD, Olsen EA, Whiting D, et al (1998) Finasteride in the treatment of men with androgenetic alopecia. J Am Acad Dermatol 39:578–589
2. Leyden J, Dunlap F, Miller B, et al (1999) Finasteride in the treatment of men with frontal male pattern hair loss. J Am Acad Dermatol 40:930–937
3. Kaufman KD, Rotonda J, Shah AK, et al (2008) Long term treatment with Finasteride 1 mg decreases the likelihood of developing further visible hair loss in men with androgenetic alopecia. Eur J Dermatol 18:400–406
4. Price VH, Menefee E, Sanchez M, et al (2006) Changes in hair weight in men with androgenetic alopecia after treatment with finasteride (1 mg daily): 3- and 4-year results. J Am Acad Dermatol 55:71–74
5. Kawashima M, Hayashi N, Igarashi A, et al (2004) Finasteride in the treatment of Japanese men with male pattern hair loss. Eur J Dermatol 14:247–254
6. Lin JH, Chen WC (2002) Finasteride in the treatment of Taiwanese men with androgenetic alopecia: a 12-month open-label study. Kaohsiung J Med Sci 18:379–385
7. Savin RC (1987) Use of topical minoxidil in the treatment of male pattern baldness. J Am Acad Dermatol 16:696–704
8. Connors TJ, Cooke DE, De Launey WE, et al (1990) Australian trial of topical minoxidil and placebo in early male pattern baldness. Australas J Dermatol 31:17–25
9. Kuan YZ, Chen SY, Chen MJ, et al (1990) Safety and efficacy of 2% topical minoxidil in the management of male pattern baldness in the Chinese. Changgeng Yi Xue Za Zhi 13:96–103

10. Olsen EA, Dunlap FE, Funicella T, et al (2002) A randomized clinical trial of 5% topical minoxidil versus 2% topical minoxidil and placebo in the treatment of androgenetic alopecia in men. J Am Acad Dermatol 47:377–385
11.Stough D (2007) Dutasteride improves male pattern hair loss in a randomized study in identical twins. J Cosmet Dermatol 6:9–13
12. Olsen EA, Hordinsky M, Whiting D (2006) The importance of dual 5-alpha-reductase inhibition in the treatment of male pattern hair loss: results of a randomized placebo-controlled study of dutasteride versus finasteride. J Am Acad Dermatol 55:1014–1023
13. DeVillez Rl, Jacobs JP, Szpunar CA, et al (1994) Androgenic alopecia in the female. Arch Dermatol 130:303–307
14. Dawber RPR, Rundegren J (2003) Hypertrichosis in females applying minoxidil solution and in normal controls. J Eur Acad Dermatol Venereol 17:271–275
15. Tsuboi R, Tanaka T, Nishikawa T, et al (2007) A randomized, placebo-controlled trial of 1% topical minoxidil solution in the treatment of androgenetic alopecia in Japanese women. Eur J Dermatol 17:37–44
16. Lucky AW, Piacquadio DJ, Ditre CM, et al (2004) A randomized placebo-controlled trial of 5% and 2% topical minoxidil solution in the treatment of female pattern hair loss. J Am Acad Dermatol 50:541–553
17. Sinclair R, Wewerinke M, Jolley D (2005) Treatment of female pattern hair loss with oral antiandrogens. Br J Dermatol 152:466–473
18. Avram MR, Cole JP, Gandelman M, et al (2002) The potential role of minoxidil in the hair transplantation setting: roundtable consensus meeting of the 9th annual meeting of the International Society of Hair Restoration Surgery. Dermatol Surg 28:894–900
19. Roenigk HH, Berman MD (1993) Topical 2% minoxidil with hair transplantation. Face 4:213–216
20. Leavitt M, Perez-Meza D, Rao NA, et al (2005) Effects of finasteride (1 mg) on hair transplant. Dermatol Surg 31: 1268–76
21. Roy RK, Thakur M, Dixit VK (2007) Development and evaluation of polyherbal formulation for hair growth-promoting activity. J Cosmet Dermatol 6:108–112
22. Adhirajan N, Ravi Kumar T, Shanmugasundaram N, et al (2003) In vivo and in vitro evaluation of hair growth potential of *Hibiscus rosa-sinensis* Linn. J Ethnopharmacol 88:235–239
23. Roy RK, Thakur M, Dixit VK (2008) Hair growth-promoting activity of *Eclipta alba* in male albino rats. Arch Dermatol Res 300:357–364
24. Rho SS, Park SJ, Hwang SL, et al (2005) The hair growth-promoting effect of *Asiasari radix* extract and its molecular regulation. J Dermatol Sci 38:89–97
25. Parks WS, Lee CH, Lee BG, et al (2003) The extract of *Thujae occidentalis* semen inhibited 5-alpha-reductase and androchronogenetic alopecia of B6CBAF1/j hybrid mouse. J Dermatol Sci 31:91–98
26. Kwon OS, Han JH, Yoo HG, et al (2007) Human hair growth enhancement in vitro by green tea epigaloocatechin-3-gallate (EGCG). Phytomedicine 14:551–555
27. Qian BC, Chen J, Xu HJ (1994) Pharmacological action of 101-B hair regeneration extract on skin and hair in experimental animals. Zhonqquo Zhong Xi Yi Jie He Za Zhi 14:227–229, 198.

Is There a Place for Oral Minoxidil? An Overview

D. Pathomvanich

At the regional workshop in Yokohama, Japan, in April 2007, a question was raised regarding the effectiveness of minoxidil tablets in promoting hair growth. I shared my experience in the use of this drug, and one of the attendants, the late Dr. James Arnold, urged me to disclose the information to other hair surgeons [1].

Clinical Pharmacology

Minoxidil is a peripheral vasodilator used officially as an antihypertensive. It occurs as a white crystalline powder and is soluble in alcohol and propylene glycol and slightly soluble in water. The chemical name is 2,4-pyrimidine-diamine, 6-(1-piperidinyl)-, 3-oxide. Its molecular formula is C9H15N50 with a molecular weight of 209.25.

More than 90% of the drug is absorbed from the gastrointestinal tract, reaching the maximum plasma level within the first hour and declining rapidly thereafter. The average half-life in humans is 4.2 h. Approximately 90% is metabolized predominantly in the liver by conjugation with glucuronic acid, with some by conversion to more polar products. All metabolites are excreted in the urine.

Minoxidil is a direct-acting peripheral vasodilator capable of reducing both elevated systolic and diastolic blood pressure. It does not interfere with the vasomotor reflexes and is therefore unlikely to produce orthostatic hypotension. The primary use is for the treatment of hypertension. Dosage is usually 2.5–100 mg per day as a single dose for adults.

Side Effects of Oral Minoxidil

Salt and Water Retention

Swelling of the hands, feet, lower legs, or face and rapid weight gain can occur.

D. Pathomvanich and K. Imagawa (eds.), *Hair Restoration Surgery in Asians*
DOI 10.1007/978-4-431-99659-0_15, © Springer 2010

Cardiovascular Effects

Chest pain, hypotension, and fast or irregular heartbeat are possible effects.

Hypertrichosis Without Virilism

Elongation, thickening, and increased pigmentation of fine body hair are seen in about 80% of users, developing within 3 to 6 weeks after starting therapy. Hypertrichosis is usually first noticed on the temples, glabella, forehead, or along the sideburns. Later it may extend to the back, arms, legs, and scalp. Upon discontinuation of minoxidil the growth of new hair is arrested, but 1 to 6 months may be required to resume pretreatment appearance. No endocrine abnormalities have been found to explain this abnormal hair growth.

Other Effects

Thrombocytopenia, nausea, and vomiting are uncommon. Breast tenderness occurs in less than 1%. Allergic rashes; blurred vision; flushing of the skin; headache; decreased sexual desire or impotence; lightheadedness; numbness or tingling in the hands, feet, or face have all been reported.

Contraindication

Minoxidil should not be used in pheochromocytoma or those who are sensitive to the components of the preparation. It may produce pericardial effusion and occasional tamponade. Angina pectoris may be exacerbated. Full details of the drug usage and side effects may be found in the PDR.

Minoxidil may pass from mother to child through breast milk. Therefore, women who are breastfeeding should not use minoxidil.

Role in Treating Alopecia

Topical Minoxidil

The occurrence of hair growth and hypertrichosis prompted Upjohn to further research. The drug was made into 2%–5% solutions for topical use and sold under the trade name Rogaine. It was initially marketed for men but later extended to women. The result, however, is unpredictable. Twice-daily application of the solution is time consuming and causes irritation to the scalp. The scalp at times may be stained by the white crystal residual and become oily. The new foam preparation seems to reduce the incidence of irritation but is not yet available worldwide. Recent reports showed that the foam is somewhat less effective that the liquid form.

Oral Minoxidil

For the past 16 years I have prescribed low-dose minoxidil in its oral form to a selected group of patients with advanced hair loss who are poor candidates for surgery. They did not respond to finasteride plus minoxidil in lotion form but wanted to do something to improve their appearance other than wearing a hairpiece. We followed these patients, who have reported minimal side effects. We monitored one patient twice a day for the period of 1 month and did not observe any change in blood pressure or heart rate or effects other than an increase in hair growth.

Overall, we observed more significant hair growth with oral dosage than after the use of the topical preparation. Although topical minoxidil has been reported to work mainly on the crown, those taking the tablets also observed significant hair growth in the front. When replacing the oral minoxidil tablet with the topical 5% lotion, the patients failed to gain or maintain hair growth. According to our experience, whether oral minoxidil was used alone or in conjunction with finasteride did not seem to make any significant difference in terms of results.

Many hair clinics are selling products containing minoxidil alone or combined with other ingredients such as vitamins, trace minerals, protein, biotin, amino acids, and finasteride as a special hair-growing formulation.

What is the optimal dosage to maximize hair growth but with minimal side effect? I learned from another physician, who had prescribed minoxidil extensively to treat alopecia, that 5 mg daily was enough to stimulate hair growth without any effect on blood pressure and heart rate. We have been using 5 mg daily for years despite observing that even with a lower dose, such as a 2.5 mg tablet per day or 5 mg every other day, some patients still reported significant hair growth.

The most common side effect we have observed was puffy eyelids and leg swelling. Similar to any other form of hair growth products, the gained hair will be shed in 3 to 4 months on stopping the pill. This oral form should not be used by women because it will cause hypertrichosis. This increase of facial and body hair will make patients unhappy, especially as the hypertrichosis may persist in some cases even on discontinuing the drug.

One must be reminded that the U.S. Food and Drug Administration (FDA) did not approve the use of oral minoxidil for hair growth, and it should not be considered as the first-line treatment or for routine use. However, I have seen and witnessed many patients who took this drug on their own having excellent results and with minimal side effects. I have limited the use to a small group of patients as

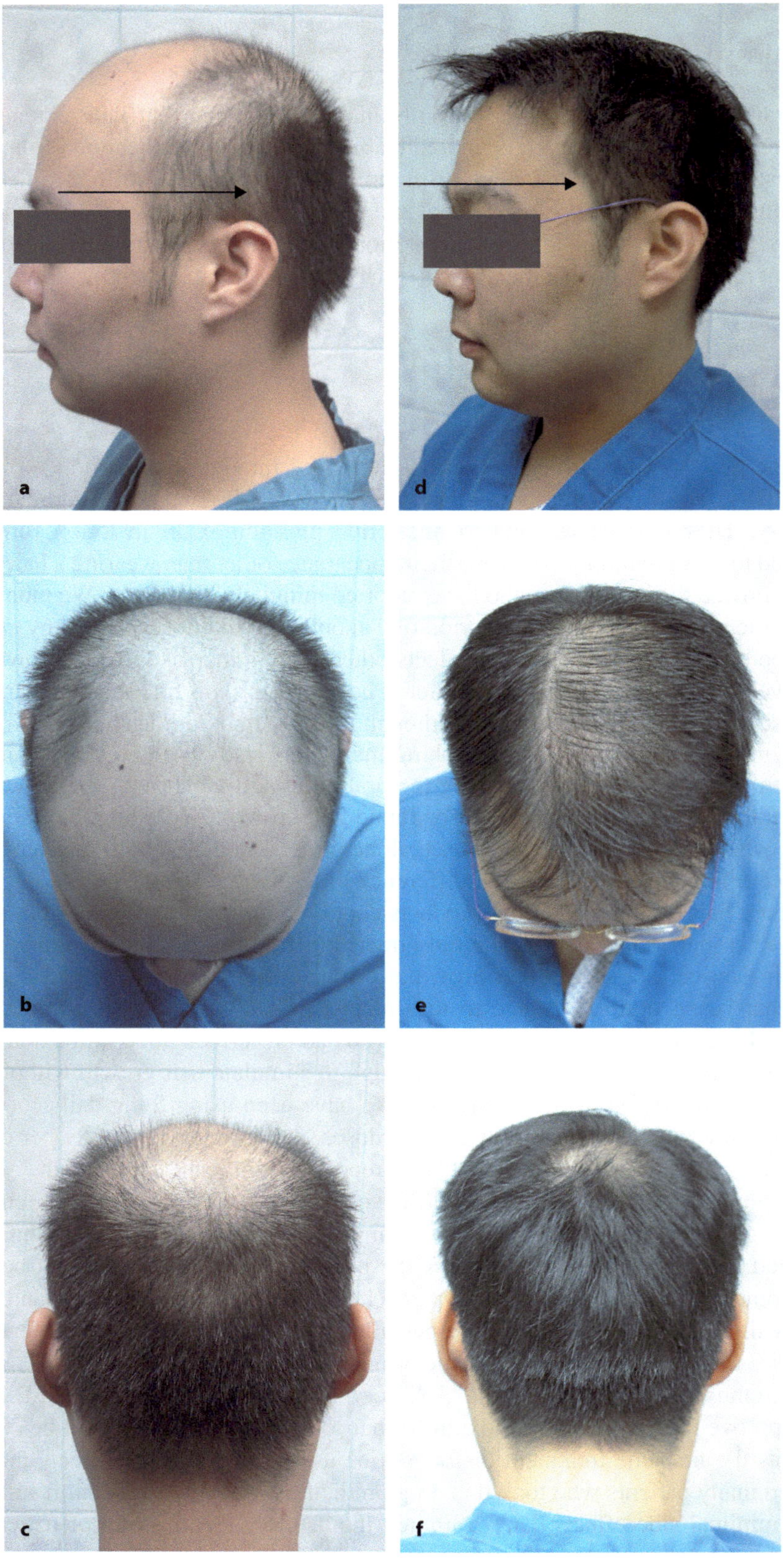

Fig. 1. **a–c** Preoperation photos. **d–f** Postoperation 2 years after 1654 FUG were transplanted + oral minoxidil, note the hair growth on both temples from minoxidil effect made poor candidate become a candidate for hair transplantation

mentioned. The majority are happy with the result and are willing to stay on the medication. A small percentage has to stop the drug after developing puffy eyelids and leg swelling. The patient must be informed of the risks and side effects and must understand that it has to be taken for life to control progressive hair loss.

As we know, no drug is absolutely safe, and any kind of medication carries some kinds of risk. So, given the risks and side effects, does the psychological impact of hair loss justify the use of minoxidil tablets?

Case Report

A 26-year-old man was seen with extensive hair loss in a very young age and wanted as much coverage as possible. 1654 FUG from limited donor supply were transplanted to the front to frame his face and he was placed on oral minoxidil post op. He has good growth of hair both temples and crown from minoxidil that enhance the result of hair transplantation (Fig. 1).

Reference

1. Arnold J (2007) Review of the ISHRS Regional Workshop: Asian Hair Surgery Workshop hosted by Kenichiro Imagawa, MD. Hair Forum Int 17:94

Part V
Preoperative Care

Preoperative Care for Super Mega-Sessions

J. Wong

In addition to the routine preoperative interview and examination, we need to emphasize three points to prepare the patient for a 3000+ grafting session.

1. The scalp needs to be in best possible shape for graft insertion; therefore, drugs such as aspirin, anticoagulants, or anything that may increase bleeding should be stopped usually 10 days preoperatively. Although there are differing views, our experiences have shown that the use of minoxidil can make graft insertion difficult, and we recommend stopping minoxidil 4 to 5 weeks preoperatively.
2. For people with poor to average laxity, stretching exercises are needed to loosen the scalp before surgery. Because Asian hair is less dense, these stretching exercises are extremely important to maximize the width of a donor strip that may be removed and closed with ease. Donor strip width is determined by the available scalp laxity, and scalp laxity can be improved with preoperative stretching exercise. To increase scalp laxity the patients are instructed to place the palm of the hands firmly on their donor area above their ears and push the scalp up and down, stretching the scalp over the bony skull. The palms must be placed firmly enough so that they do not slide over the skin surface. The donor scalp at the back is also stretched in a similar manner, using both palms with the fingers interlocked. Patients are instructed to stretch 10 to 20 times daily, working the scalp for 5 to 10 min each time. These exercises are described on our website at www.hassonandwong.com. From experience we have found that if patients do these exercises effectively, the increased donor yield can be anywhere from 500 to 1500 follicular units. People with tight scalps generally require 4 to 8 weeks to effectively stretch out their scalp, and a follow-up visit to check laxity before booking surgery is a good idea.
3. Nearly all patients undergoing sessions larger than 3500 grafts will have the recipient area shaved down to 2 mm and will need to be warned in advance as this may impact their social and work interaction for several weeks after surgery. Follicular unit transplantation (FUT) performed with precision heals very quickly, and Asians with darker skin have very little residual redness once the crusting is gone, 10 to 12 days after surgery. Most of our educated patients know about the shaving and have come to accept it, and even patients initially reluctant to be shaved are reassured after viewing postoperative photos showing how

D. Pathomvanich and K. Imagawa (eds.), *Hair Restoration Surgery in Asians*
DOI 10.1007/978-4-431-99659-0_16, © Springer 2010

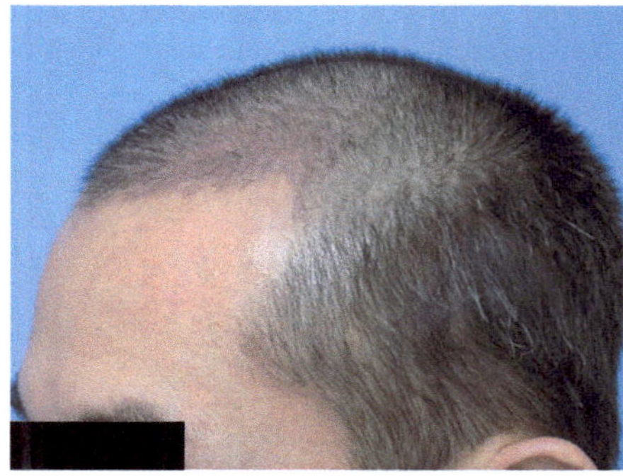

Fig. 1. At 11 days post operation with short haircut

quickly the recipient sites heal. Even with just the transplanted stubble on top there is little to show that the area has been transplanted. Most patients will be given a haircut at the time of staple removal to blend the transplanted area to the sides. It is important to remember to leave the hairs around the scar a little longer for coverage.

Part VI
Local Anesthesia and Tumescence

Safe Use of Local Anesthesia and Tumescence Fluid in the Donor Site as an Office-Based Procedure

D. Pathomvanich

It is not exaggerating to state that there are at least 100 variations in local anesthetic technique. Beginners are often confused by the wide range of xylocaine and adrenaline concentrations in the anesthetic solution and tumescence. Yet they all seem to work quite well for the individual surgeon.

Despite such diversity, there are some universally agreed-upon general principles of local anesthesia in hair transplantation.

- Use some form of premedication to allay pain and anxiety.
- Take special care with the elderly and those on other medications.
- Allow no loud noises, jokes, or chatter from staff while injecting.
- Use the finest possible needle.
- Inject slowly with freshly added adrenaline in the mix.
- Allow adequate time for hemostasis (at least 10 min).
- Top up with additional tumescence from time to time to maintain a firm cutting base.
- Re-administer additional anesthesia every 2 h in some patients.

The techniques described in this chapter are based on my personal experiences over the past 20 years.

The Safe Use of Drugs

The office's questionnaires should be used to screen patient for history of drug allergy. Before giving any injection or oral medication, the surgeon should double check if the patient had any previous reaction to local anesthetic, especially anaphylaxis or malignant hyperthermia. The surgeon should be well trained in Advanced Cardiac Life Support (ACLS) and be familiar with medications used should any complication arise.

D. Pathomvanich and K. Imagawa (eds.), *Hair Restoration Surgery in Asians*
DOI 10.1007/978-4-431-99659-0_17, © Springer 2010

Premedication

Keeping the patient well informed about the procedure with the appropriate use of preoperative sedation will reduce anxiety before entering the operating room [1]. Many approaches have been used to minimize pain in local anesthetic injection:

- Inhalation of nitrous oxide [2]
- Intravenous midazolam or propofol [3]
- Oral diazepam or midazolam
- Any combination of these

I only use oral sedation because my practice is office based. Diazepam 5–20 mg p.o. depending on patient's age, midazolam 15 mg (the oral form, which is available in Thailand and Taiwan), and a Cox II inhibitor such as Arcoxia 120 mg [4] are given one-half hour before surgery.

Drugs for Local Anesthesia

The most commonly used local anesthetic in hair transplantation is lidocaine hydrochloride. The onset of action is 2–4 min. It is rapidly metabolized from the liver, and less than 10% is excreted unchanged in the urine. Anesthesia can last up to 1 h for plain lidocaine and up to 2 h when epinephrine is added.

The maximum bolus dose for plain 1% lidocaine is 300 mg (30 ml), and 500 mg (50 ml) when combined with epinephrine. For a super mega-session that lasts up to 8–12 h, infiltrating the recipient site with a larger dose of lidocaine is needed to eliminate pain during insertion.

Bupivacaine (Marcaine) 0.25% when compared to lidocaine has a slower onset of action (5–10 min). Its anesthetic effect, however, lasts longer, up to 4 h. Infiltration of bupivacaine is very painful, but the main drawback is its irreversible cardiotoxic effects, manifested as arrhythmia and fibrillation.

The maximum single dosages for plain bupivacaine is 175 mg, and 225 mg when combined with epinephrine 1 : 200,000 [5]. Injection can be repeated every 3 h, not exceeding a total of 400 mg in any 24 h.

Despite its potential cardiotoxic side effects, bupivacaine is still widely used by many cosmetic surgeons (PDR 60th edition, 2006). It should however be avoided in patients with cardiac conditions.

Previously I used both bupivacaine and lidocaine in hair transplantation. As no difference was observed in the duration of their anesthetic effect, the use of bupivacaine was abandoned from fear of its side effects. Currently I use only lidocaine with epinephrine and continue to search for longer-acting agents for use in mega-sessions.

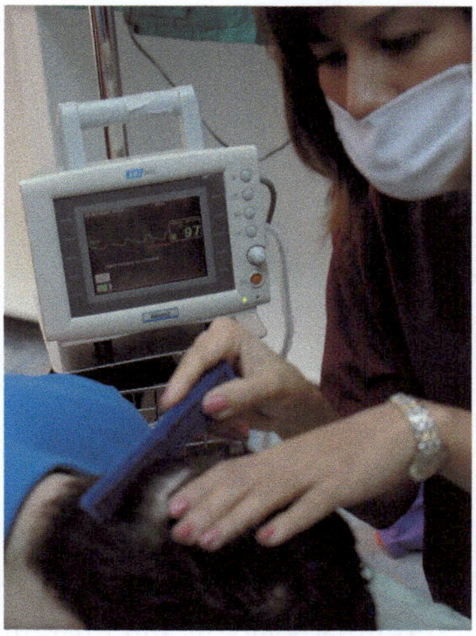

Fig. 1. Monitoring with pulse oximetry

Monitoring

During the entire injecting procedure, the blood pressure, heart rate, and oxygen saturation should be monitored. Pulse oximetry is the minimal requirement (Fig. 1), and EKG should be used if available. At any time when the monitor signals tachycardia, I stop injecting immediately, and only resume when the rhythm returns to normal.

Personal Techniques

Some recommend applying eutectic mixture of local anesthesia (EMLA) 3% or benzocaine [6] to the area 2 h before injection. Rand slow drip is favored by some, but the process is time consuming and the machine is expensive [7,8]. Desensitizing the area with ice cubes or a small vibrator [9] just before injection has produced good results. Massage is another good means of distraction (Fig. 2).

There are three steps in preparing the donor site.

1. Intradermal wheal: Three to four evenly spaced wheals, about 1 cm below the strip, are first raised by very slow intradermal injection [10]. The smallest size 30 G needles are used to minimize pain. I routinely use 0.5% lidocaine with 1 : 300 000 epinephrine. Buffering with sodium bicarbonate (9 : 1 ratio) has been shown to further reduce patient discomfort [7,11]. Premixed lidocaine with epinephrine is not recommended as it is adjusted to a lower pH (3.5–5) to prolong half-life, and the acidity causes more discomfort on injection [12,13].

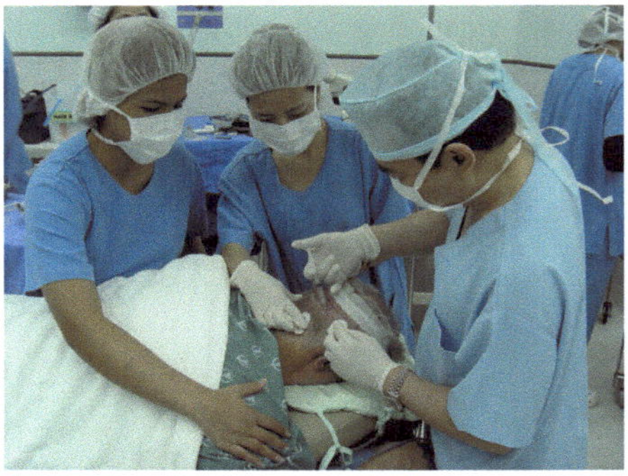

Fig. 2. Massage as a form of distraction when injecting local anesthesia

2. Local anesthetic infiltration: 27 G needles are reinserted via the anesthetized skin, advancing and injecting the same solution slowly in both directions. Two to three assistants can inject simultaneously to save time. This process is repeated until the entire inferior border is anesthetized. On average a total of 4–8 ml is adequate to provide a painless working field.
3. Tumescence: My tumescent fluid is composed of 0.1% lidocaine with epinephrine 1 : 250 000–1 : 500 000. It should be injected at least 2–3 cm beyond the upper and lower margins of the incision. On average a large quantity (50–150 ml) is required to achieve long-lasting anesthetic and hemostatic effects. Alternatively, the tumescent can be injected first via the three or four anesthetized intradermal wheals. On completion, the entire donor strip is then topped up with 0.5% or 1% lidocaine. When the two options were compared, I found the first method faster and less painful.

In the elderly and patients with cardiac conditions, the lowest concentration of epinephrine should be used in tumescence, only topped up with a higher concentration in case of excessive bleeding. I reserve 30 ml tumescent fluid to be injected later as my refined open technique requires more time and attention to minimize graft transection. Surgeons who can complete the strip excision within a short period of time should inject all tumescence before harvesting.

The operative area is then painted with betadine and draped, ready for the surgeon.

References

1. Larson CP (1992) Evaluation of the patient and preoperative preparation. In: Barash PG, Cullen BF, Stoelting RK (eds) Clinical anesthesia. Lippincott, Philadelphia, pp 545–562
2. Sadick N, Stough D (1996) Nitrous oxide in hair restoration surgery. In: Hair replacement: surgical and medical. Mosby, St. Louis, pp 104–105
3. Abeles G (1999) The combined use of propofol and fentanyl for outpatient intravenous conscious sedation. Dermatol Surg 25:599–562

4. Parsley W (2004) Management of the postoperative period. In: Unger WP, Shapiro R (eds) Hair transplantation, 4th edn. Dekker, New York, pp 555–568
5. Seager D (1996) Local anesthesia in hair transplantation. In: Hair replacement: surgical and medical. Mosby, St. Louis, pp 81–89
6. Ginzburg A (2004) Tips for the hair transplant surgeon. Hair Transplant Forum Int 14(2)
7. Barusco M, Leavitt M, Heathrow R (2001) The use of a computerized anesthesia injection system to minimize pain during hair transplant surgery. Hair Transplant Forum Int 11(4)
8. Epstein J (2001) Commentaries on Barusco's use of a computerized anesthesia injection system to minimize pain during hair transplant surgery. Hair Transplant Forum Int 11(4)
9. Wolf BR (2004) Anesthesia. In: Unger WP, Shapiro R (eds) Hair transplantation, 4th edn. Dekker, New York, pp 225–247
10. Hanke W, Sommer B, Sattler G (1998) Tumescent local anesthesia 2001, Medical. p 212
11. Palmon SC, Lloyd AT, Kirsch JR (1998) The effect of needle gauge and lidocaine pH on pain during intradermal injection. Anesth Analg 86:379–381
12. Wong J (2005) Lateral, dense, mega—is this the future? Hair Transplant Forum Int 15(1)
13. Field LM, Namias A (1999) Bilevel tumescent anesthetic infiltration for hair transplantation. Dermatol Surg 25:152

Preparing for a Painless Surgery: Medication or Meditation?

J. Wong

Premedication

Having been trained by Dr. Mario Marzola of Australia at the beginning of my transplantation career, I adopted his routine of IV sedation using midazolam and fentenyl before local anesthesia. Subsequently, if patients do feel the pain of injection at the time, they do not remember it as a result of the amnesic effect of the midazolam. Dr. Marzola always said "Don't hurt the patients or they won't come back," and in the early days of my practice all the patients were transplanted under heavy sedation.

In those days, when the average session size was 400 grafts, it was important for patients to come back multiple times to slowly build up coverage and density. Two years after starting my hair practice, a policy change by our provincial college made it impractical to use IV sedation, and patients did find the local injections very painful. Many patients have commented that if it were not so painful they would have come back for a second procedure.

Today there are several methods to make the injections more tolerable, and the one I like best involves the use of a small vibrator and a dental injector (Fig. 1). Although this method does not eliminate the pain of injections completely, most people find the injections quite tolerable. In most of the cases, we do not use preoperative sedation unless the patient is extremely nervous. If needed, 5 to 10 mg diazepam p.o. is given before the start of surgery, and this dose is usually sufficient to calm the patient during the strip removal and site preparation. Because patients are only lightly sedated, he (or she) is still able to cooperate with changing and holding different head positions for strip removal and is also able to get up and move about for periodic stretch breaks.

For the occasional patient who has a real fear of needles and requires more sedation, 2 mg midazolam i.m. may be given. This drug will act over the next several minutes, producing a nice calming effect without overly sedating the patient. For the past 15 years we have not required any intravenous sedation or sedatives.

One of the most common causes of fainting spells during surgery is hypoglycemia. Instruct the patient to eat before surgery, also give them some juice or a light snack after strip removal, and always provide and insist that they eat lunch and

D. Pathomvanich and K. Imagawa (eds.), *Hair Restoration Surgery in Asians*
DOI 10.1007/978-4-431-99659-0_18, © Springer 2010

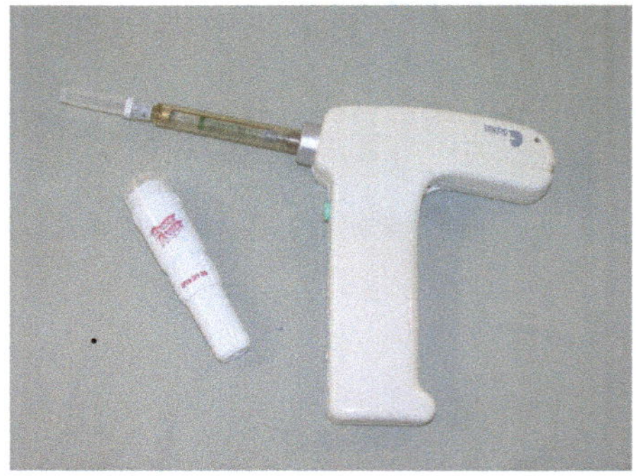

Fig. 1. Vibrator and dental injector

supper if the surgery runs into the evening. We also find television is a very helpful distraction for the patient during long procedures. To prevent deep vein thrombosis, have the patient get up for a quick stretch every 60 to 90 min.

Short- and Long-Acting Local Anesthetic

The typical length of the donor strip for a mega session is 29 to 31 cm; therefore, we need a fairly quick and efficient method to numb a very wide area. Time management is critical as sessions can sometimes take as long as 10 to 12 h. The donor site is numbed using 1% xylocaine with adrenalin. To start I make ink dots with a surgical marker spaced 2 cm apart 1 cm below the donor area. Two to three drops of xylocaine is then injected into each dot using a 30 G needle while at the same time a small vibrator is applied to the skin below the injection site to act as a distraction. If the area has significant scar tissue from previous surgery, change the needle at the first sign of dullness.

The vibrator combined with slow injection will greatly reduce the pain for most patients, and once the initial 1–2 drops of xylocaine is deposited the dotted areas are partially numbed. A second round of xylocaine can be injected into the exact same area using more pressure and volume. A third round of xylocaine injected between the dots ensures total numbness; on average, this requires a total of 9 to 12 ml 1% xylocaine. If there are scars from previous surgery, more local is required. For the majority of patients 1% xylocaine is sufficient and will provide anesthesia for approximately 3.5 h. At 3.5 h after the start of surgery, the donor area is topped up using 0.25% marcaine with adrenalin. The top-up is usually painless as the area is still numb and will provide a further 7 to 10 h of anesthesia. Only occasionally does anyone require further topping up. The key here is to wait 3.5 h after the initial injection (of xylocaine) before giving the marcaine, thus making maximum use of both local anesthetics.

The front is done in the same fashion, but because the front is more sensitive than the back, the initial injections for the line block is done using the Dentro injector set at low speed for the initial round. The Dentro injector uses 2% xylocaine ampules with 1 : 200 000 adrenalin and a 33 G needle. Because the injector controls the flow rate and keeps it very slow, it is far less painful than a hand syringe. The Dentro injector holds 2 ml 2% xylocaine, which is enough to numb the dotted areas along the line block. Additional 2% xylocaine is then injected using a 10 cc syringe and a 30 G needle until total anesthesia is obtained.

Occasionally there may be an area in the front that is difficult to anesthetize that may respond to very superficial injections in the dermis. The first round of anesthetic will usually last 3 to 4 h, and if top-ups are required, 2% xylocaine may be used. In individuals in whom the anesthetic wears off quickly requiring multiple top-ups, 0.25% marcaine may be used. Because the graft insertion starts from the front and proceeds back, one top-up is generally all that is required.

Part VII
Donor Harvesting

Site Selection in Donor Harvesting: A Long and Winding Road

D. Pathomvanich

Successful hair transplantation is often limited by the available donor hairs. It is logical to minimize hair follicle transection during harvesting to ensure an optimal result.

Most methods for donor harvesting [1] are blind techniques. The follicular papillae are not visualized on dissection. One such technique is the use of multi-bladed knives. Although this method shortens harvesting time, the blades unavoidably damage many hair follicles along their course [2]. Some transected hair follicles may continue to grow. However, the quality of these hairs is often poor [3,4].

The occiput is quite irregular in topography. Here the hair follicles are rooted in random depths and directions. Any slight deviation of the scalpel or punch cutting angle will result in transection.

One current method in minimizing such transection is to incise parallel to the donor hair shafts [5]. Still, one is guessing at the angles of the follicles in a single dimension. The significant difference in their alignments renders it virtually impossible to parallel the blade along the hair shafts.

Dissection of follicles around previous strip scars is even more challenging. Their directions are often distorted, particularly along the inferior side.

Donor Site Selection

Hair loss is progressive and unpredictable. One major concern in hair restoration surgery is how to harvest permanent hairs from the safe donor area without compromising supply for subsequent sessions. Harvesting beyond the safe donor area may create a wide scar and pick up nonpermanent hairs [6]. Such a mistake is easily made when selection is made too high, or when a young patient presents with early hair loss. What appears to be the "safe hair" today might become "unsafe" in the future. When hair loss advances with age, this coarse hair may become finer with each cycle [7].

To predict the pattern of future hair loss, the family history of alopecia on both maternal and paternal sides *must* be assessed during the initial consultation.

D. Pathomvanich and K. Imagawa (eds.), *Hair Restoration Surgery in Asians*
DOI 10.1007/978-4-431-99659-0_19, © Springer 2010

Obviously, this will not help if no one else in the family is bald, or the patient was adopted, not knowing the biological parents. The new genetic test for androgenic alopecia [8] that was designed to predict the susceptibility might be helpful but will not contribute to knowing the extent and progress of hair loss.

Defining the Donor Area

Stough and Haber first selected the lowest part of the safe donor site for the first session. During subsequent sessions the new strip is taken above but not including the previous scar. Stough later changed to his refined donor harvesting technique. The incision was started laterally at the parietals and then extended to the mid-occiput; this was to make use of the parietal hair in early procedures [9].

I select the donor hair by first assessing the extent of hair loss and availability of donor hair. The patient must be seated in good lighting with wet hair. The good old rule of thumb was to start at the nuchal ridge. From experience, however, this is not always practical as in some patients the thinning area may well pass below the nuchal ridge.

Alt and Unger have written extensively regarding the "safe donor area" [5]. In class III to V it is good practice to use the superior nuchal ridge as a landmark. The incision can start here, where good-quality hairs are usually found, and extend bilaterally to both auricles. The family history of hair loss must be kept in mind in these groups.

In class VI to VII it is better to search for good-quality hair and mark the upper and lower safe margins between the superior parieto-occipital rim and the nape of the neck. *The area halfway between the good fringes is then harvested.* For a patient with a large temple projection and good-quality temporal hair, I may start from the pre-auricle 3 cm behind the good hair at the temple point. In the older age group with a poor quality of hair it is better to stop at wherever good hair diminishes. In some patients, this may be behind the ears (Fig. 1).

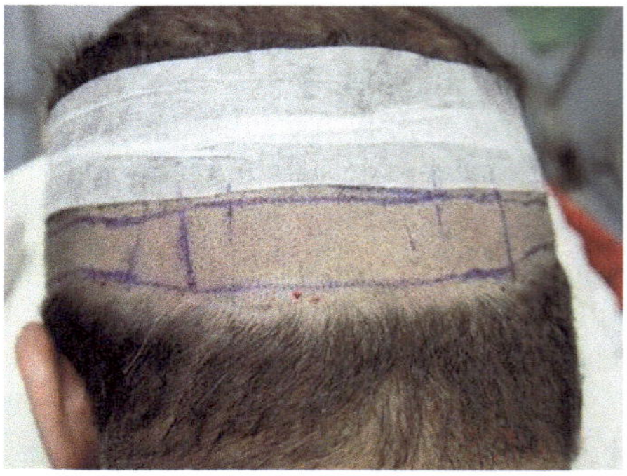

Fig. 1. Defining the donor strip

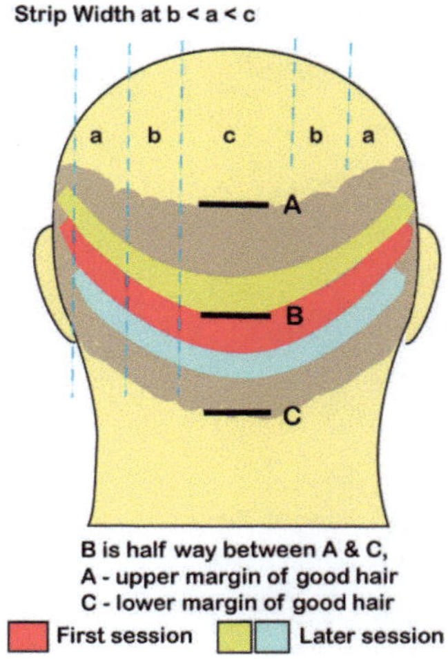

Fig. 2. Marking the donor strip in a mega-session

Mega-Session

A large quantity of hair is needed for a mega-session. The strip has to be from one pre-auricle to the other pre-auricle. For a subsequent mega-session, if the previous donor scar is small, I mark the inferior strip margin at least 1.0 cm above this old scar. It would be difficult to include an old scar where the hairs are intermingled and distorted in direction. Transection can be high even with careful dissection [5]. Even if a new scar is created it should be minimal and acceptable if the incision is closed by a trichophytic closure in the majority of patients.

Some patients may be concerned about having too many scars. The previous scar can then be included as one margin or within the incised strip. Because hair density is low within the scar, the number of grafts will be less (Fig. 2).

Small Session

When selecting the strip for the first procedure, one must plan for future sessions. If only a minimal to moderate number of grafts is required, I start at the mid-occiput and extend into both parietals. A future strip can be selected in the same area. The previous scar can be included to leave just one linear scar [6].

If more sessions are anticipated in the future, I extend the incision from the mid-occiput to the left auricle. Any previous scar will be included at its inferior margin. The right parietal can then be preserved for future harvesting.

It is more difficult to mark a strip for those who already had multiple sessions. Many wide scars are expected and some may even crisscross each other. It is better not to include any scar. First, the hair along the previous incision is usually fine,

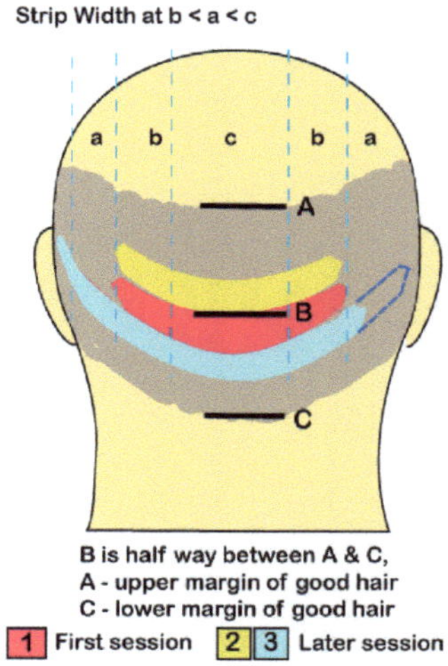

Fig. 3. Defining the donor strip in a small session

probably a combined effect of transected follicles and reduced vascular supply. Moreover, including scars will further reduce the number of grafts. In a class VI patient this is insufficient for any cosmetic improvement.

Patients who had punch grafts in the past would have reduced density by at least 50% in the parieto-occipital region The temporoparietal area in many is usually still virgin on both sides and should provide a reasonable number of grafts (Fig. 3).

Preoperative Scalp Massage

If performed properly, preoperative scalp massage will loosen any tight scalp [10]. This is essential especially in those with previous surgery or scalp reduction. A minimum of 15 to 20 min two to three times a day, or a total of 200–300 lifts, is recommended. Scalp exercise should commence at least 4 to 6 weeks before surgery. The patient very often will notice improvement in laxity after 2 weeks.

Step-by-Step Scalp Massage

1. Press the heel of both palms flat and firmly onto the hair-bearing scalp above the ears.
2. Lift the scalp up as much as possible and hold this hand position for 10 s by counting “one” to “ten.”
3. Move and work toward the occipital region.
4. Cross fingers in both hands and lay the locked palms onto the scalp on approaching the occiput.

A donor site should be selected carefully. The transplantation of permanent hair that looks good after many decades and the minimization of scars in the donor area reflect the ability of the hair transplant surgeon.

References

1. Unger W, Cole J (2004) The donor area. In: Unger WP, Shapiro R (eds) Hair transplantation, 4th edn. Dekker, New York, pp 301–304
2. Rose P, Shapiro R (2004) Combining microscopic slivering with backlighting and loupe magnification to efficiently produce grafts. In: Unger WP, Shapiro R (eds) Hair transplantation, 4th edn. Dekker, New York, pp 365–367
3. Kim J, Choi Y (1995) Regrowth of grafted human scalp hair after removal of the bulb. Dermatol Surg 95:312–313
4. Beechner M (2004) Studies of hair survival in grafts of different sizes. In: Unger WP, Shapiro R (eds) Hair transplantation, 4th edn. Dekker, New York, pp 261–279
5. Unger W, Cole J (2004) The donor area. In: Unger WP, Shapiro R (eds) Hair transplantation, 4th edn. Dekker, New York, pp 301–304
6. Stough D, Haber R (1996) The donor site. In: Hair replacement: surgical and medical. Mosby, St. Louis, pp 132–123
7. Unger WP, Shapiro R (2004) The initial interview. In: Unger WP, Shapiro R (eds) Hair transplantation, 4th edn. Dekker, New York, pp 165–176
8. Keene S (2008) A genetic test for androgenetic alopecia: polymorphisms in the androgen receptor gene provide a genetic screening test for androgenetic alopecia and earlier medical intervention. Hair Forum Int 18:91
9. Stough DB, Haber RS (1996) The donor site. In: Stough DB, Haber RS (eds) Hair replacement: surgical and medical. Mosby, St. Louis, pp 131–132
10. Swinehart J (1996) Preoperative preparation and haemostasis. In: Color atlas of hair restoration surgery. Appleton & Lange, East Norwalk, CT, pp 123–132

The Strip: How Long, How Wide, and Where?

D. Pathomvanich

Instead of guessing, as most hair transplant surgeons have done in the past, the length and width of the donor strip should first be calculated using the following methods.

Recipient Area and Desired Number of Grafts

The area to be transplanted should be measured before surgery. There are many methods to estimate the bald area. The Fargo method is based on projection of geometric shapes such as a square, rectangle, circle, or triangle onto the recipient site. Geometric formulas are then used to summate the total surface area [1].

The method described by Chang is simple and easy to apply [2]. A clear plastic sheet such as Saran wrap is first attached to a large embroidery plastic ring. Alternatively, the wrap can be stretched and directly laid over the recipient area. The outer margin of the bald area is outlined with a fine marker [3]. The marked wrap is then transferred onto a metric scale containing boxes of 1 cm^2. One method is to count the intersections in the grid using the principle of morphometrics, and the number of intersections will closely approximate the areas inside the tracing in centimeters squared [4]. However, for an accurate estimation counting the actual number of blocks is preferred (Fig. 1).

For a given desired recipient site density, the number of grafts (N) required is determined by the formula:

$$\textit{Desired density } (D) \times \textit{total recipient area } (A)$$

Different clinics will have their own protocols concerning the desired density. For example, if D is 40 follicles/cm^2 and the total recipient area (A) is 50 cm^2, the number of grafts (N) required is $40 \times 50 = 2000$.

It is important to discuss with the patient before deciding on how many follicular units (FUs) to be transplanted in one session, or in two or three sessions. This number will depend not only on the amount of donor hair available but on how

D. Pathomvanich and K. Imagawa (eds.), *Hair Restoration Surgery in Asians*
DOI 10.1007/978-4-431-99659-0_20, © Springer 2010

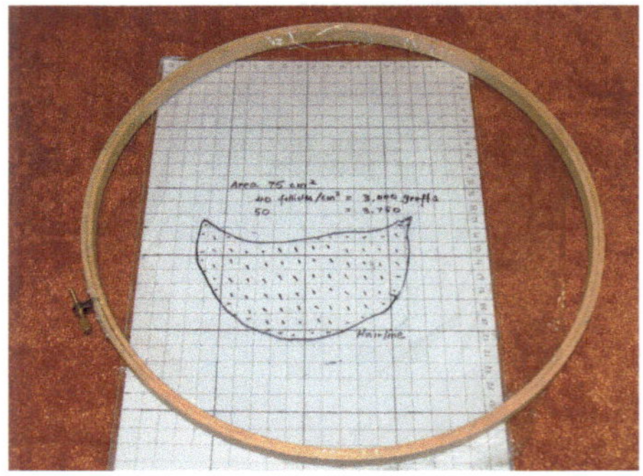

Fig. 1. Counting the number of 1 cm^2 blocks

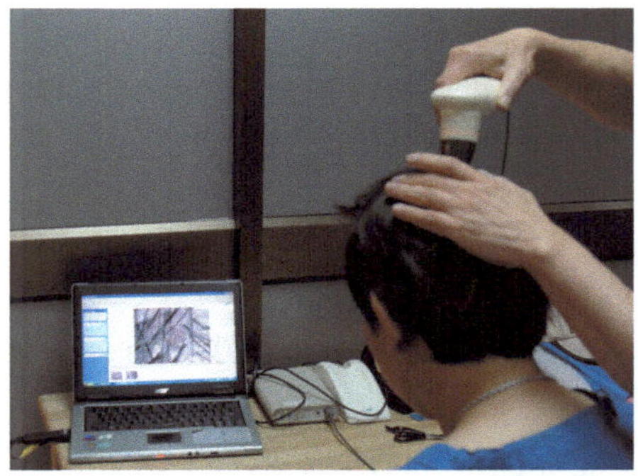

Fig. 2. A Trichoscan

much hair the patient wants and how much he or she can afford to pay. However, the new trend is toward one pass if possible in the good candidate.

Hair Count

Hair count can be obtained by using the Rassman densitometer, Welch Allyn trichoscope, Trichoscan (Fig. 2), etc. The Rassman densitometer is a personal preference as it is easy to make counts and the calculations compared with other devices. Unfortunately, Radio Shack is no longer producing this densitometer. Similar-looking devices may be available at some merchandise or medical supply sources at very low cost (Fig. 3).

The Trichoscan using a macro-image camera or portable USB microscope transfers the images onto a computer screen. It has the advantage that the count can be made by several observers simultaneously to arrive at a more objective result. Also, the pictures can be kept in the patient's record to compare with follow-up counts, giving evidence of hair growth after transplantation.

The hair must be trimmed short to make accurate count of the following:

1. The number of hairs
2. The number of follicular units

Fig. 3. A look-alike densitometer

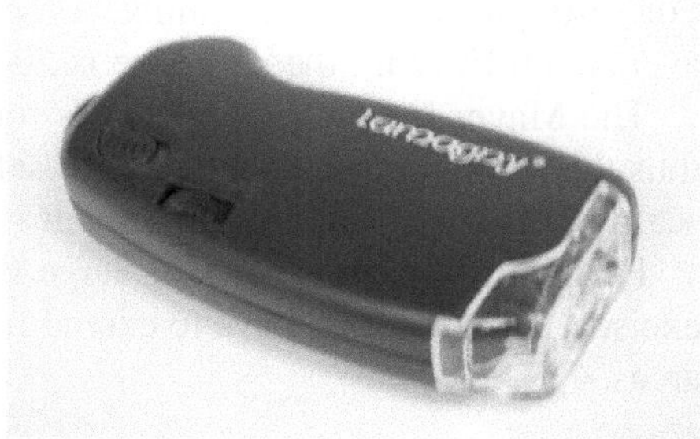

3. The number of miniaturized hairs
4. The ratio of one-, two-, and three-hair follicular units

The information is important in preparing pre-made incisions and predicting the outcome of surgery. Too many single-hair FUs (see ratio of FU by Imagawa) and miniaturized hair will have poor outcome.

Sometimes it is difficult to determine if a bunch of hair is, say, two 1-hair FUs or one 2-hair FU. Any misinterpretation will lead to a discrepancy in the final number. It is helpful to ask the graft-cutting assistants to make the count.

One common problem encountered is that gray or white hair is difficult to visualize and count on direct inspection. Gentian violet and methylene blue have been used in the past to dye the hair but this is messy and not really effective. The best solution is to have the patient color the hair the night before surgery or, preferably, have the hair colored before surgery at a salon. Emphasize to the hair stylist the need to make sure the color stains the hair close to the scalp. There are many hair-coloring products available on the market. An instant hair coloring preparation works quickly and is the best do-it-yourself choice. For those patients reluctant to have their hair dyed, permission should be granted to apply black mascara to the short stumps of gray or white hair just in the harvesting area.

As hair density varies throughout the donor area, we used the method described by Cole [5] in our clinic to arrive at an average reading (*B*). Cole recommended using three reference points to make a count on a long strip (mid-occipital protuberance, above the ear, and a point halfway in between). For a short strip he used one single point over the mid-mastoid area, but I generally prefer taking two reference points for a more accurate reading. The miniaturized hair is not counted in calculating the strip size.

Strip Size and Width

The strip size (*S*) is calculated as follows:

$$S = \textit{Total number of grafts required } (N) \div \textit{Average density } (B)$$

For example, if the total number of grafts required is 2000, and donor density average 80 FU/cm^2, the strip size is 2000 grafts divided by 80 = 25 cm^2.

The Mayer [6] scaling method is routinely used to assess the scalp laxity and thus the maximum width that can be safely excised. I found it is reliable on virgin scalp but less accurate on subsequent sessions.

For a super mega-session, a large donor area, 40 to 55 cm^2, may have to be excised. The strip may have to extend from the mid-occiput to both supra-auricular areas.

Mid-Occipital Area

A strip 1.5 to 3.0 cm wide can be excised here depending on scalp laxity.

Mastoid

The laxity here is usually less. A narrow strip, 1.0 to 1.5 cm, has to be used to ensure minimal tension in closure.

Supra-Auricular Area

Here in many patients a wider scar is observed than at the mid-occiput, even when the scalp laxity and strip width are the same. The width should therefore be slightly less, around 1.5 to 2.5 cm. There are two possible explanations: in this region, the scalp contains three instead of five layers; or the excision cuts across Langer's line [7–9]. In some individuals, this area cannot be used as the hair is too fine and low in density to cover any strip scar.

Marking the Strip

When outlining the strip area, a fine-point marker should be used. Scoring along the upper or lower margin of a thick line would affect the number of grafts. A caliper is a good option. Its pair of sharp points can be dipped in gentian violet after the calculated width is accurately set between the arms. To ensure drawing a very thin line, the hair must be trimmed very short and the skin should be wiped dry (Fig. 4).

One option is to apply pre-cut firm plastic templates of different sizes (e.g., 1.0 × 30 cm^2, 1.5 × 15 cm^2, 2.0 × 15 cm^2). Tracing along the templates is quick

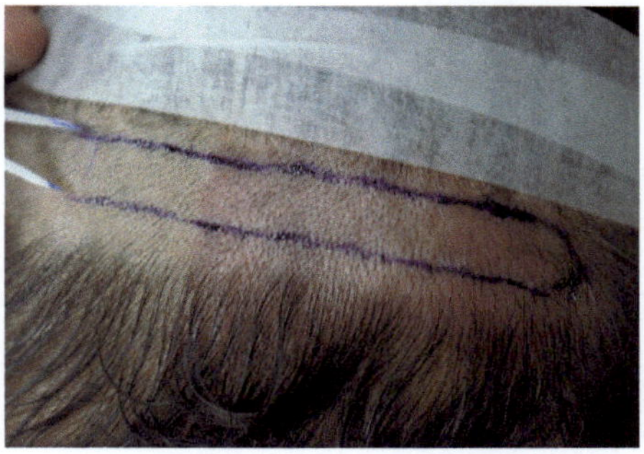

Fig. 4. Marking a strip

but it sometimes leaves marks blurred with ink, so a good-quality marking pen is needed.

Another simple method is to mark the desired width along the donor area with dots 3 to 4 cm apart and then join them together.

References

1. Farjo B (2001) Estimating graft numbers made easy for the recipient site. HT Forum Int 11:101
2. Chang S (2001) Estimate number of graft and donor area. HT Forum Int 4:97–102
3. Pathomvanich D (2006) Hair transplantation in Asians. In: Haber RS, Stough DB (eds) Hair transplantation. Elsevier Saunders, Philadelphia, pp 149–155
4. Parsley W (2006) Follicular unit instrument. In: Haber RS, Stough DB (eds) Hair transplantation. Elsevier Saunders, Philadelphia, pp 99–109
5. Cole J (2004) Donor harvesting. In: Unger W, Shapiro R (eds) Hair transplantation, 4th edn. Dekker, New York, p 306
6. Mayer M (2005) Scalp elasticity scale. HT Forum Int 15(4)
7. Gerry SE. Surgical anatomy of the scalp. In: Unger W, Shapiro R (eds) Hair transplantation, 4th edn. Dekker, New York, pp 37–41
8. Gerry SE (2001) Galea fixation. Dermatol Surg 27:931–936
9. Gerry SE (2002) Surgical anatomy of the scalp. Dermatol Surg 28:581–587

A Refined Open Donor Harvesting to Minimize Follicular Transection

D. Pathomvanich

Strip excision is by far the most common method currently used for donor harvesting in hair restoration surgery throughout the world [1–6]. Although there are many different techniques in strip excision, almost all are blind techniques. The surgeon's skill and experience are required in keeping the scalpel blade parallel to the hair shaft to minimize transection. What appears to be a straight hair may have the root curved in an unpredictable direction. Hair follicles are arranged not in orderly but in random rows. Even hairs in the same follicle may be found in different planes and angles. The worst scenario is obviously the curly hair where it is impossible to parallel the blade with the hair shaft. Hair transection during blind cutting is inevitable.

Asian hair usually has longer and coarser follicles and, together with a thick scalp, the potential for transection during harvesting is high. To overcome this, Arturo Sandoval described his "triple S" technique [7] in which he used clamps to spread open the incision after scoring. The author reported the open technique in *Hair Forum International* in October 1998 [8], and subsequently in the journal *Dermatologic Surgery* in April 2000 [9]. It was difficult to describe the technique in detail on paper, however, and hands-on experience and close observation were required to appreciate its merit. For the past 10 years, I have refined the technique for easy and speedy harvesting.

Instruments

Only simple instruments are required including four skin hooks, a 3–4× magnifying loupe, Swanz Morton or Personna Plus blades (no. 15 and 10), and a small suction device. The patient lies prone on a prone pillow.

Preparation and Technique

The strip size is calculated as described in another chapter and outlined with a very fine point marker. The hair must be trimmed as close to the scalp as possible along

D. Pathomvanich and K. Imagawa (eds.), *Hair Restoration Surgery in Asians*
DOI 10.1007/978-4-431-99659-0_21,

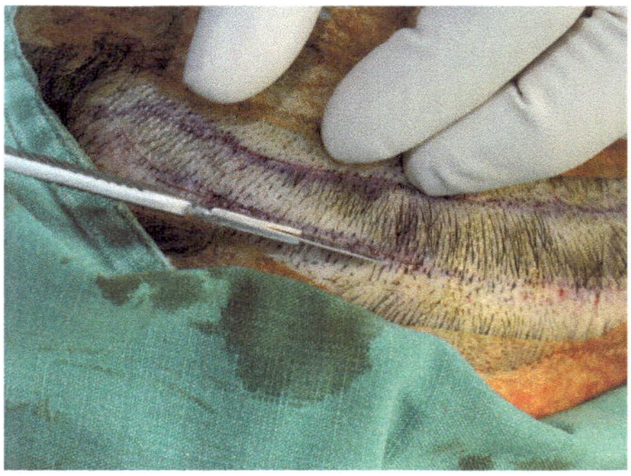

Fig. 1. Scoring

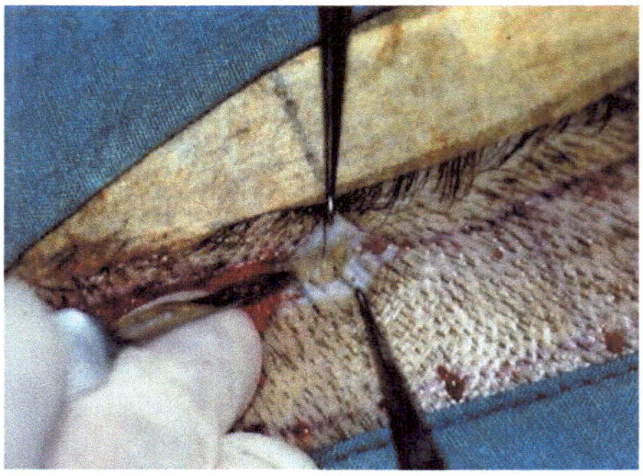

Fig. 2. Two skin hooks

the incision because there is no need to see and follow hair direction. The area is then infiltrated with 0.5% lidocaine with epinephrine followed by tumescent fluid. I prefer 0.1% lidocaine with epinephrine 1 : 250 000 for the elderly. Epinephrine is diluted further to 1 : 500 000 for those with cardiovascular problems. For effective hemostasis, the tumescence fluid has to be injected repeatedly during harvesting as the fluid disperses very rapidly. The incision is scored superficially with a number 10 blade along the fine line. Scoring too deeply will transect the follicles (Fig. 1).

Skin hooks are then applied to the exposed superficial dermis on each side of the incision for fast and "open" dissection. The number of skin hooks will depend on the number of assistants available:

Two skin hooks: positioned on opposite sides of the incision (Fig. 2).
Three skin hooks: two on one side and the other positioned in between on the opposite side forming a triangle (Fig. 3).
Four skin hooks: described by Dow Stough [10] with two skin hooks on each side (Fig. 4).

The skin hooks must be checked and adjusted to ensure they catch only the upper or mid-dermis and not the follicles. They are then lifted and pulled in opposite directions. Constant traction must be maintained while running the blade. Care

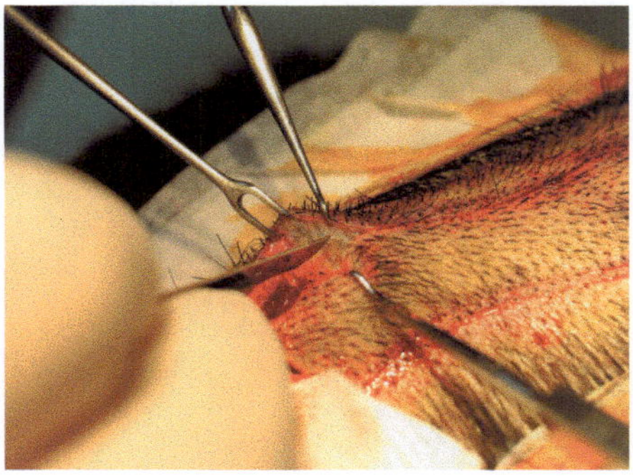

Fig. 3. Three skin hooks

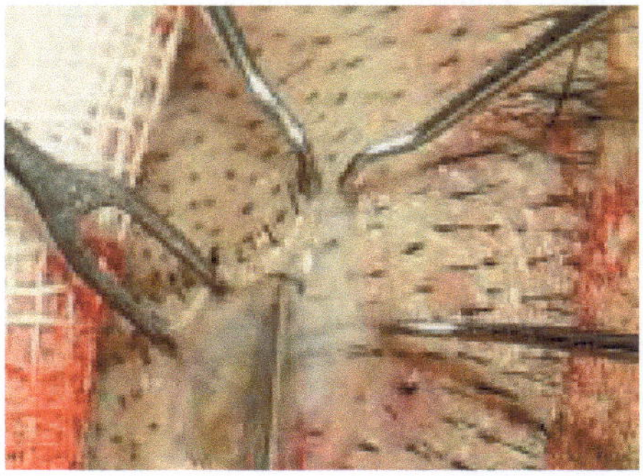

Fig. 4. Four skin hooks. Note that an entire follicle lies across the incision

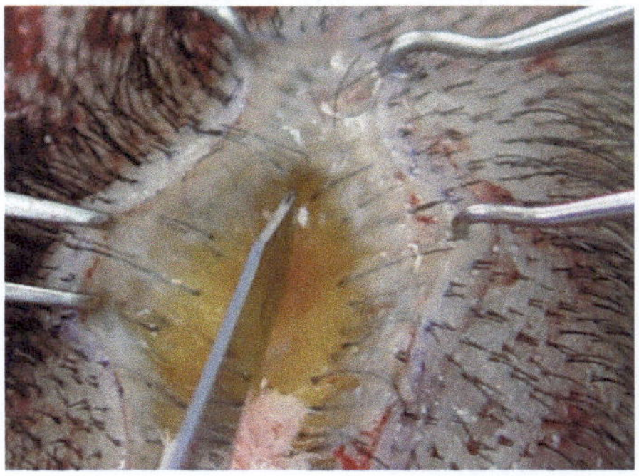

Fig. 5. Dissecting down to dermal papilla

should be exercised to dissect between the follicles and open the incision down to the dermal papilla (Fig. 5).

There are many strategies for dissection. The sharp tip of the blade is a powerful tool. One can strike the tissue between the follicle with the pointed tip (Fig. 6), keeping it parallel to the hair shaft during cutting. Besides slivering, the belly of the blade can also be utilized to touch and cut the tissue when there is no follicle found on the scored incision.

During the course of dissecting the surgeon may encounter the following:

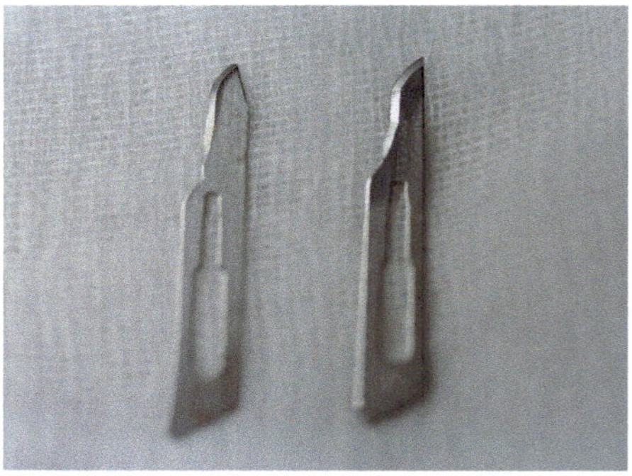

Fig. 6. The sharp tip of no. 15 blade (Swann Morton and Personna)

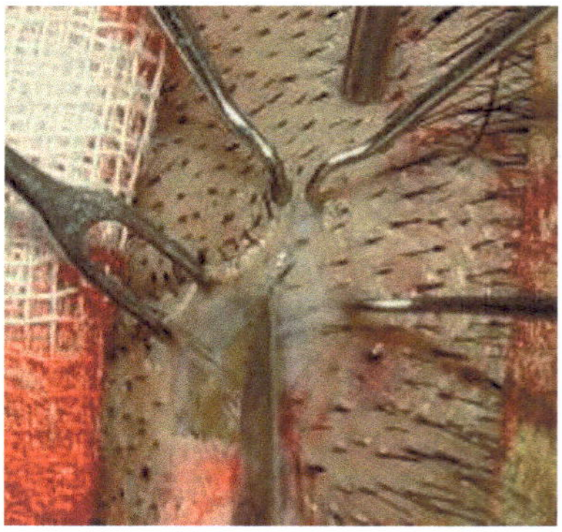

Fig. 7. Follicle located in the middle of the incision

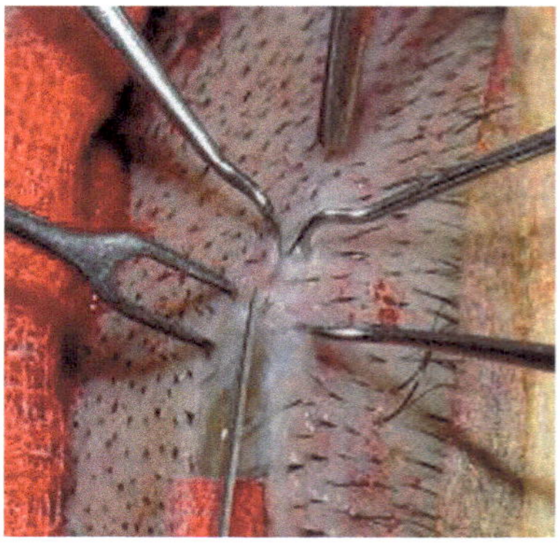

Fig. 8. Follicle located close to either side of the incision

1. The entire follicle lies across the incision (see Fig. 4),which increases the potential for transection. The follicle can be pulled and tipped to one side using a skin hook or the dull part of the blade tip.
2. The follicle is located in the middle of the incision (Fig. 7). One can easily dissect on either side of the follicle. If more grafts are needed, the follicle should be included into the strip.
3. The follicle is located close to either side of the incision (Fig. 8). Here careful dissection will spare all the follicles from unnecessary damage.

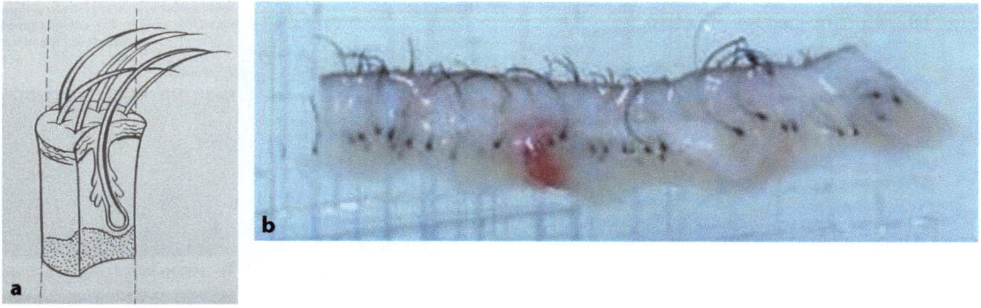

Fig. 9. C-shaped follicles

The surgeon has to identify the position of the oncoming follicle and keep track of the blade before cutting to avoid transection. If the hairs are very dense and the roots interlock with each other, there is no need to cut all the way down to the dermal papilla. Gentle traction on the skin hook can easily open up the incision so long as the area contains no scar. For fast track one can dissect halfway for 1 to 2 cm before returning for deep dissection. As mentioned previously, tumescent fluid must be reinjected to reassure hemostasis during cutting. The use of a small suction tip will free the incision of all blood for clear dissecting.

The dissecting technique may have to be adjusted to cater for the different curvatures of hair.

1. Straight hair is straightforward as described.
2. For curly hair, as in Afro-Americans, the dissection is much easier because the density is lower than that of the Caucasian with a greater distance between follicles. Also, the entire follicles do not stay deep in the subcutaneous layer as seen in Asians. The C-shape of the follicle creates some concern among surgeons. James Arnold [11] suggested bending the blade to match the curvature of the hair follicle to reduce transection (Fig. 9). However, it is not easy to bend the blade to match the curly hair as the blade is often broken during manipulation. From our experience, the curling follicle can be easily straightened up on lifting with the skin hook.
3. Gray hair is difficult because the follicles cannot be visualized: no matter what technique is used, dissection is still blind. I score slightly deeper and use skin hooks to separate the incision. The blade touches the tissue without forceful cutting. If the follicle is cut, one can feel the friction as if cutting grass.

Dividing the Strip

Once a length of 7 to 10 cm is reached on both sides, the first piece is removed by cutting underneath the strip with a number 10 blade. The strip should be held under traction and wrapped by wet gauze to prevent desiccation. It is safer to first cut on

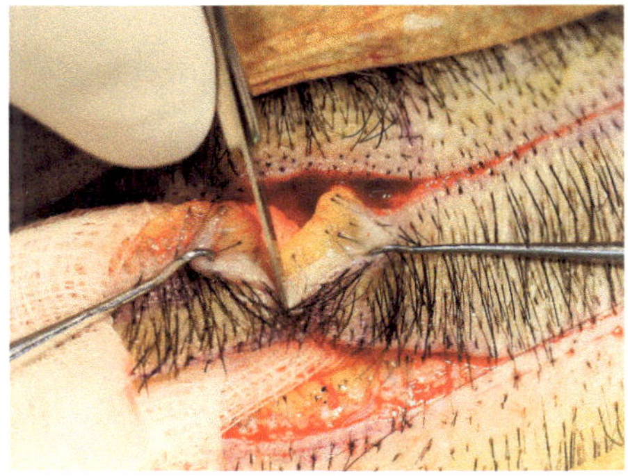

Fig. 10. Cutting across the strip

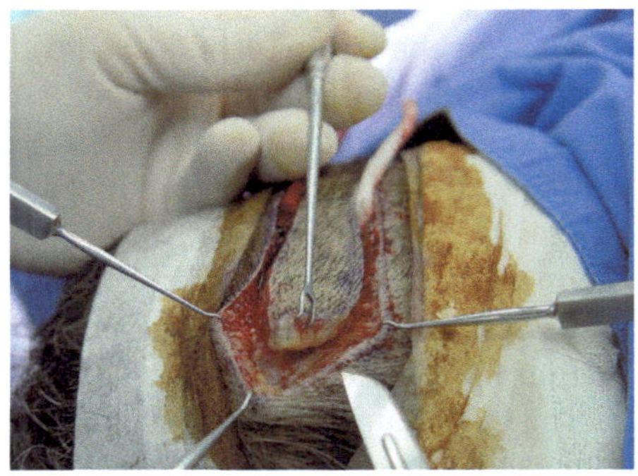

Fig. 11. Dissecting the tip of the strip

each side of the strip with the roots on view in freeing the strip. Directly cutting the base of strip may lacerate the dermal papilla, so beginners must be careful.

To remove the strip, two skin hooks are gently applied 1 cm in front of the undissected margin to avoid back-bleeding. Minimal pulling force should be employed, just to stabilize the strip. Using only the tip of the blade to cut across between follicles, the strip is then divided (Fig. 10), ready for microscopic dissection.

If bleeding is minimal, the incision is packed with wet saline gauze. The lower flap is routinely de-epithelialized before dissecting the rest of the strip in the same fashion. In case of bleeding, 3/0 nylon is used to approximate the wound. These retention sutures can achieve hemostasis, reduce tension at the wound edges, and facilitate later wound closure.

The end of the strip has the highest potential for transection as the incision changes from linear to curvilinear (Fig. 11). The assistants should apply two or three skin hooks to both sides or tip of the incision. At the same time the surgeon pulls and lifts up the strip using skin hook or fingers, dissecting the tip just below the dermal papilla.

For a super mega-session (3000+ grafts), the strip is dissected completely. However, instead of taking the whole strip out to sit around for another 6–7 h, only the first half of the strip is removed. The other half is removed 3–4 h later to increase graft survival. When this last strip is removed, tumescent fluid has to be reinjected at its middle to decrease bleeding. The entire incision is then closed with interrupted 3/0 nylon retention stitches followed by 4/0 rapid vicryl running or layer closure. Although by this time the local anesthetic is still effective, it should be reinjected after wound closing. Some surgeons might use nonabsorbable stitches or skin staples as their preference.

My experience with retention stitches is that these always have a smaller scar compared with layer closure or single layer stitches that I have used in the past. However, most surgeons are still using layer closure for wide strip excision with or without undermining.

R. Haber introduced a spreader for fast harvesting [12]. I do not have experience with this spreader, but personal communication with K. Imagawa and W.-Y. Wu indicates they were not happy with using the device for Asians and no longer use this instrument.

References

1. Unger W (1995) The donor site. In: Unger W (ed) Hair transplantation. Dekker, New York, pp 183–212
2. Rassman W, Carson S (1995) Micrografting in extensive quantities. Dermatol Surg 4:306–311
3. Nordstrom EA (1995) An alternative method of evaluating efficacy of technique. In: Unger W (ed) Hair transplantation. Dekker, New York, pp 67–68
4. Bernstein R, Rassman W (1999) The logic of follicular unit transplantation. Dermatol Clin 17:277–295
5. Haber R, Stough D (1996) Accurate estimation of grafts requirements when using multi-blade knives. In: Haber RS, Stough DB (eds) Hair replacement: surgical and medical. Mosby, St. Louis, pp 138–142
6. Limmer BL (1996) Elliptical donor stereoscopically assisted technique. In: Haber RS, Stough DB (eds) Hair replacement: surgical and medical. Mosby, St. Louis, pp 133–137
7. Parsley W (2005) Pioneer of the month: Arturo Sandoval Camarena, MD. Hair Transplant Forum 15(6)
8. Pathomvanich D (1998) Donor harvesting, a new approach to minimizing transection of the hair follicle: Hair Transplant Forum 8(5):1,4–5
9. Pathomvanich D (2000) Donor harvesting: a new approach to minimize transection of hair follicles. Dermatol Surg 26:345–348
10. Stough DB (2006) Tension donor harvesting. Video in Haber R, Stough D (eds) Hair transplantation. Elsevier Saunders, Philadelphia
11. Arnold J (2002) Harvesting donor tissue in African-Americans. Cyberspace Chat. Hair Transplant Forum 12(4)
12. Mayer M (2006) Report on Haber spreader technique at European Society of Hair Restoration Surgery: 9th Annual Congress and Live Surgery Workshop. Hair Transplant Forum 4(127)

Other Methods of Donor Harvesting

D. Pathomvanich

We are all aware that hair follicles are not always arranged parallel or in rows. There are variations in hair direction and angles over the scalp. This deviation is most obvious at the cowlick, where hairs exit as a swirl. Fortunately, a cowlick is not often found at a donor site. Also, the shaft exiting from the scalp does not necessarily follow the same angle as the infundibulum. In many people the donor hair, instead of pointing inferiorly, may be directed sideways either to the left or to the right. Consequently, any harvesting technique carries a risk for transecting these follicles. The different hair directions in the donor site must be examined properly before harvesting.

The punch graft was first used by Okuda [1], a Japanese dermatologist, back in 1939. This method became popular when Orentreich used a similar hand punch 4–5 mm in diameter in treating male pattern hair loss (MPHL) and later published his work in 1959 [2]. At present I believe no one would use a large punch of this size for donor harvesting. The use of a motorized trephine subsequently allowed faster and more uniform plug creation (Fig. 1). However it had numerous disadvantages, including slow healing of the donor sites, which were not sutured before around 1980. This method resulted in circular white scars and sometimes a cobblestone appearance when there was any hypertrophy in the healing. Later the plugs were excised very close together in a process called "strip-punching" and the defect sutured. The use of the mechanized punch rapidly declined after it was recognized that acquired immunodeficiency syndrome (AIDS) was caused by a blood-borne virus and that blood was atomized by the rapidly spinning punch.

The single-bladed knife was first described by Coiffman [3] and was popularized by Uebel [4] and Limmer [5] in excising the donor strip. The transection rate was low, as reported by Limmer at 3%–5% [5] and Cole at 2%–4% [6], making it an attractive method when compared with the punch grafts as mentioned. The number 10 blade is used more often than the number 15 blade, and it should be held parallel to the hair shaft on incising. Some surgeons such as Carlos Uebel cut with the belly of the blade as one stroke deep down to the fatty tissue. Most surgeons hold the knife perpendicular to the skin, trying to stay parallel to the hair shaft. Others prefer holding the blade at a 45° angle. The strip must be checked each few centimeters and the angle of the blade adjusted if transection is encountered.

D. Pathomvanich and K. Imagawa (eds.), *Hair Restoration Surgery in Asians*
DOI 10.1007/978-4-431-99659-0_22, © Springer 2010

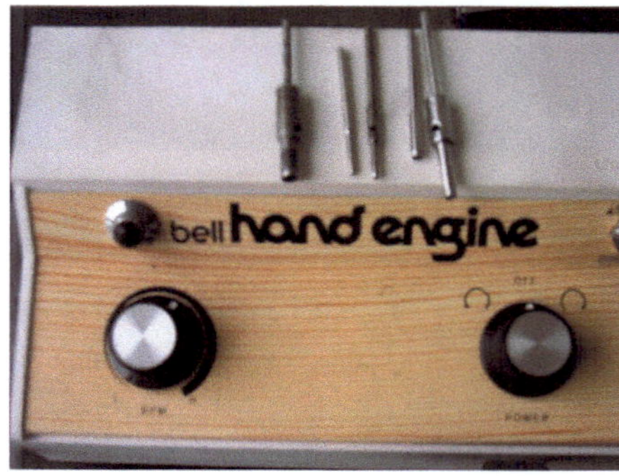

Fig. 1. Hand engine used in the past for punch grafts harvesting

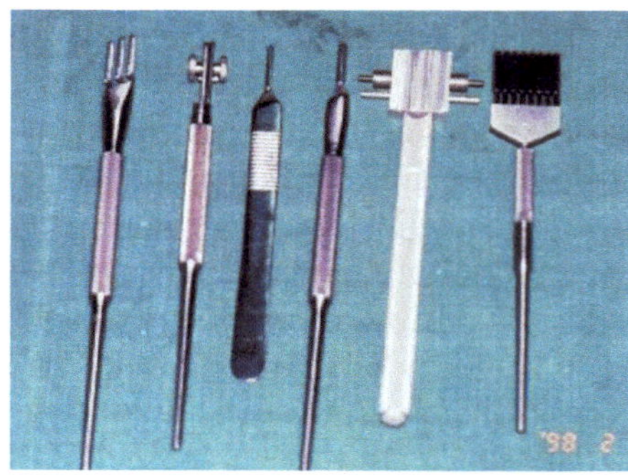

Fig. 2. Different types of multi-bladed knife

Kadach [7] proposed her "Roots? Angle up. No roots? Angle down" theory. However, by the time you adjust the blade, follicular transection has already occurred. The technique is fast and is still used by the majority of hair surgeons. It is a blind technique, and the transection rate is unpredictable, especially in curly hair; obviously it would be less in experienced hands. Incising the first side of the strip usually produces less transection because of scalp tension. After one side is freed, the strip becomes loose and flaccid. Transection is therefore higher when cutting the remaining side.

Multi-bladed knives have been used since 1968 (Fig. 2). Vallis first reported using a double-bladed knife for donor harvesting [8]. Emil Bisaccia and Dwight A. Scarborough [9,10] introduced the triple-bladed knife in 1990. Subsequently more blades were advocated, and Pascal Boudjema [11] used up to six to harvest multiple narrow strips. Grafts are then cut from the strips by using a microtome and press. This technique has many advantages. First, it is fast and easy to master. Multiple strips of equal size can be obtained at the same time, reducing the slivering time. Fewer assistants are required in cutting, yet a large number of grafts can be obtained in less than 1 h. This method is therefore still favored by many hair transplant surgeons.

Mangubat [12] used up to nine blades to obtain multiple narrow strips. The strips are then laid on his grafts cutter device. By using impulsive force, grafts of uniform size can be obtained in a short period of time. The main drawback is its very high transection rate, as reported by Rassman [13]. This technique is no longer used by the majority of hair surgeons.

Multi-blades when cutting multi-strips will increase the number of strip surfaces. Griffin suggested in Ref [14] that the total transection rate can be calculated by multiplying the number of transection on one surface with the number of blades. There are a variety of blade handles, and catalogues can be obtained from vendors such as Robbins, Ellis Instruments, and A-Z instruments.

I used multi-bladed knives in the early 1990s. Different type of handles and approaches were tried to overcome the difficulties in harvesting the Asian scalp. Eventually this technique was abandoned because of the unacceptably high number of transections. I would not recommend its use in an Asian scalp. However, double-bladed knives can still be used for superficial scoring.

Follicular unit extraction (FUE) is another method of donor harvesting. It was first pioneered by Dr. Ray Wood from Australia, but his personal technique remains a secret. This method is discussed further in Dr. Bertram Ng's chapter on FUE.

The automated hair transplant system by using an automatic punch machine is outlined in Dr. Imagawa's chapter.

Robotic-assisted harvest of follicular units is being developed by a medical device company, the Restoration Robotic Inc. An image-guided robotic system is designed for hair transplantation, and the system is currently undergoing clinical testing. The reported transection rate is still high at 6%–13% [15] but is much improved when compared with 30% [16] reported a year ago at the 16th Annual Scientific ISHRS Meeting in Las Vegas.

In summary, hair transplant surgeons must understand and learn all the methods of donor harvesting that are available today, and then use their own judgment to decide what techniques should be used to minimize the transection rate as low as possible, and to produce more grafts and reduce donor scars.

References

1. Okuda S (1939) Clinical and experimental study of living hair transplantation. Jpn J Dermatol Urol 46:6
2. Orentreich N (1959) Autografts in alopecias and other selected dermatological conditions. Ann N Y Acad Sci 83:463
3. Coiffman F (1977) Use of square scalp grafts for male pattern baldness. Int J Plast Reconstruct Surg 60:228–232
4. Uebel CO (1991) Micrografts and minigrafts: a new approach for baldness surgery. Ann Plast Surg 27:476–487
5. Limmer BL (1996) Elliptical donor harvesting. In: Stough D, Haber R (eds) Hair replacement: surgical and medical. Mosby, St. Louis, pp 142–144
6. Cole J (2004) Donor harvesting. In: Unger W, Shapiro R (eds) Hair transplantation, 4th edn. Dekker, New York, pp 342–344
7. Kadach D (1999) Letter to the Editor: A step toward the perfect strip... From another angle. Hair Transplant Forum Int 9:46

8. Vallis CP (1969) Surgical treatment of receding hair line. Plast Reconstr Surg 44:271–278
9. Bisaccia E, Scarborough D (1990) A technique for square plug hair transplantation. Am J Cosmet Surg 7:219–222
10. Bisaccia E, Scarborough D (1994) Hair transplant by incisional strip harvesting. J Dermatol Surg Oncol 20:443–448
11. Boudjema P (1996) Automated hair transplant system: the Boudjema technique. In: Stough D, Haber R (eds) Hair replacement: surgical and medical. Mosby, St. Louis, pp 370–372
12. Mangubat A (2004) Impulsive force grafts preparation. In: Unger W, Shapiro R (eds) Hair transplantation, 4th edn. Dekker, New York, pp 372–379
13. Rassman W (1998) Blind graft production with cutting grates and multi-bladed knives. Hair Transplant Forum Int 8(5):22–23
14. Unger W, Cole J (2004) Donor harvesting: excision of donor strip. In: Unger W, Shapiro R (eds) Hair transplantation, 4th edn. Dekker, New York, p 323
15. Canales MG (2008) Robotic-assisted harvest of follicular. Presentation at 16th ISHRS scientific annual meeting in Montreal, Canada
16. Canales MG (2007) Robotic-assisted harvest of follicular. Presentation at 15th ISHRS scientific annual meeting in Las Vegas, NV

Omnigraft™

K. Imagawa

There was a big dispute about the pros and cons of automation hair transplantation in the 1990s.

Automated machines mechanically made cut-to-size grafts with an impulsive force. Many hair transplant surgeons were apprehensive about the potential high risk of follicular transection (FT). We may say that the results of machines were disappointing, judged by their poor results in micro- and mini-grafting.

With time, most of the machines have faded from the market because of the entry of their strongest rival, follicular unit transplantation (FUT). However, the situation in Japan is different from Western countries. There are still big franchised clinics actively promoting the procedures using Omnigraft™, which is the successor of Calvitron™ made by the French company Medicamat. The operation system of Omnigraft™ consists of two options in harvesting:

1. Multi-bladed knife and graft cutter device (Hairtome)
2. Motor-driven punch (powered follicular unit extraction, FUE)

This step is followed by graft placement using an implantation hand piece. The system is advocated to be cost-effective by reducing operation time and the number of required staff.

However, the machines have been criticized in some aspects.

Criticism of Multi-Bladed Knife and Hairtome

The potential risk of follicular transection by a multi-bladed knife is undoubtedly higher than that of a single-bladed knife. Bernstein has condemned the use as a "holocaust of donor hair" [1]. Stough reported that the unpredictability of transection when using a multi-bladed knife was between 8% and 20%, and this figure was reached by careful evaluation under a microscope [2].

Yamamoto, who has extensive experience in Omnigraft™, frankly commented: "the combination of multi bladed knife and Hairtome produces an average follicular transection rate of 30%, leading to considerable low hair growth or thin hair after transplant. Therefore a high-quality dense-packing procedure cannot be achieved by this technique, and the machine should be used only when the team consists mainly or entirely of inexperienced staff" [3].

I agree with Yamamoto that we must always seek refined and high-quality hair transplant techniques. Rather than using this machine, however, the author suggests that inexperienced surgeons seek to improve their technique with conventional methods of hair transplantation.

Criticism of Powered FUE

In 2008, Onda et al. reported that follicular transection using 1–1.25 mm motor-driven punches attached to Omnigraft™ is 5.4%. This figure is much lower than the 17.3% by conventional manual FUEs [4]. However, Yamamoto reached totally opposite results. He reported that in his total 21 cases there was less than 30% transection in 6 cases, 30%–60% in 7 cases, and more than 60% in 8 cases using a powered punch. He also commented that manual FUE had a better score than powered FUE in difficult cases except the former was a more time-consuming technique. He concluded that powered FUE was preferred in easy cases when a

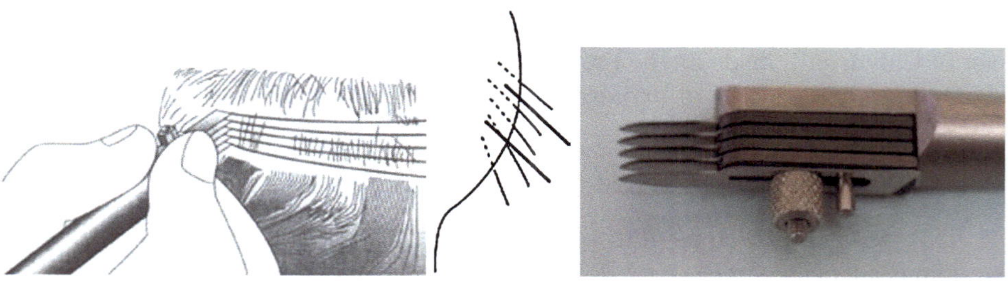

Fig. 1. Follicular transection using multi-bladed knife. Hair direction of each incision varies, and the multi-bladed knife has a potentially higher risk of follicular transection that would cause low survival and miniaturization of the donor hair

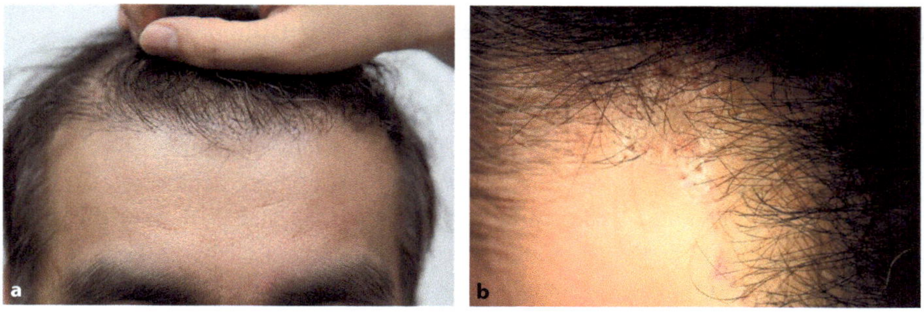

Fig. 2. Typical case done using Omnigraft. **a** Pitting is seen in most of the patients. **b** Close-up view

low transection rate was anticipated, and that manual FUE should be used in difficult cases [5,6]. Yamamoto's conclusion seems more persuasive than that of Onda. Still, knowing the very high transection rate of the device, I cannot agree with him in this issue as we must always choose the method that produces the "best result." We must remember however that experts using any technique or devise can usually obtain better results than those who only use the technique occasionally.

Criticism of Graft Replacement by Implantation Hand Piece

The micro-hole technique is definitely not as good as the micro-slit technique in dense packing; the former causes more scalp damage. Nakatsui reported that scarring made by the micro-hole technique is four times larger than that of micro-slit [7]. Actually, the hyperfibrotic scarring and severe "shock loss" is quite often observed in cases using Omnigraft™. I saw numerous bad results performed by machines, but I believe the bad results were generally a result of surgical inexperience rather than any specific fault of the machines.

Unfortunately, comprehensive information about Omnigraft™ is hard to find, and closer inspection and a structured evaluation for this procedure are still required.

References

1. Bernstein RB (1998) Blind graft production: value at what cost? Hair Transplant Forum Int 8:28–29
2. Stough DB (2006) Tension donor dissection: the ultimate strip harvesting method. Hair Transplant Forum Int 17:77–78
3. Yamamoto K (2007) Hair transplantation using Omnigraft™. J Jpn Soc Aesthetic Surg 44:106–113 (in Japanese)
4. Onda M, Igawa HH, Inoue K, et al (2008) Novel technique of follicular unit extraction hair transplantation with a powered punching device. Dermatol Surg 34:1683–1688
5. Yamamoto K (2007) Treatment of baldness by FUE. J Jpn Soc Dermatol Surg 11:110–111 (in Japanese)
6. Yamamoto K (2008) Mechanical FUE vs. manual FUE. J Jpn Soc Aesthetic Surg 45:74 (abstract in Japanese)
7. Nakatsui TC (2004) Doing away with incision length. Hair Transplant Forum Int 14:149–150

Donor Wound Closure

D. Pathomvanich

Bleeding from Wound

Hemostasis should be achieved before wound closure. I usually pack the incision with moist gauze as I dissect. When active bleeding is difficult to control, the vessel can be picked up and clamped by a pair of artery forceps. If the vessel is small the hemostat can be released before wound closure. On the other hand, if the vessel is large and at the center of incision, it is best to control the bleeding by 4/0 vicryl ligature or low-current cautery. In my practice I have to use cautery two to three times a month, so it is advisable to have the equipment.

The infrared coagulator has been used in the past to achieve hemostasis [1]. However, it has another benefit. In a study of 24 patients using a pulse duration of 2.5 s, it was noted that the wound was significantly reduced in width by an average of 42% before closure [2], which makes the wound easier to close and with minimal tension. For some reason its usage has seemed to fade away. In short, the bleeding will very often be arrested by direct pressure.

I use suction to clear the field, and irrigate the wound with normal saline to remove any tissue debris, foreign body, or fragment of hair before wound closure.

Trichophytic Closure

Asians have lower donor hairs per square centimeter and a high contrast between the usually very black hair and the white skin. The donor scar is therefore more likely to be visible, particularly with young patients who generally develop wider scars than older patients because of the higher proportion of elastic fibers in their skin.

Over the years many techniques in producing an invisible scar have been explored. The trichophytic donor closure was first introduced by Drs. Patrick Frechet, Mario Marzola, and Paul Rose in 2005 [3–6]. Marzola trimmed the lip of the superior flap before closing the wound [5].

I have used this technique for 6 months but did not observe any improvement of the scar when compared with the nontrichophytic cases [6]. I then switched to

D. Pathomvanich and K. Imagawa (eds.), *Hair Restoration Surgery in Asians*
DOI 10.1007/978-4-431-99659-0_23, © Springer 2010

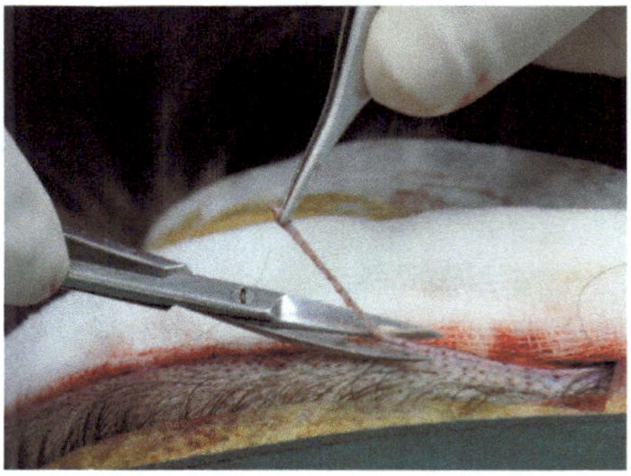

Fig. 1. Trichophytic closure (excision of lower lip)

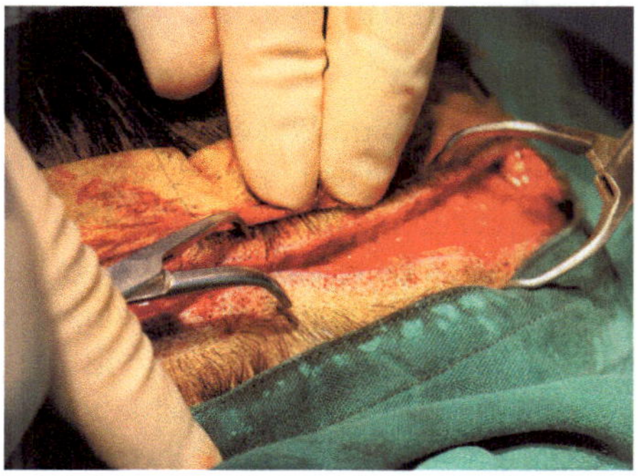

Fig. 2. Retention clamp

inferior trichophytic closure and have seen remarkable improvement in more than 80% of the cases (Fig. 1). The scars are invisible or minimal at less than 2 mm (Fig. 2).

I also found that Asian scalp skin is thick and hard. It is very difficult to trim the skin edge just with scissors. It is better to first score a 1-mm line parallel to the edge of the lower flap with a number 10 blade. A similar score is made <1 mm below the incision in a horizontal plane. The skin can then be easily trimmed away from the wound edge.

Because it is difficult to get uniform edge excision, Puig [7] described a simple tool, a double-bladed knife with a long spacer. The control depth and width are set to 1–1.5 mm. Dae-Young Kim [8] uses a 5-cc syringe as a blade handle. A bent razor is pushed into the syringe cylinder. The exposed sharp blade is then used to cut at uniform depth control.

Undermining

Patrick Frechet [3] commented that to obtain an invisible scar the maximum width of incision should not exceed 1 cm, and either the superior or inferior flap should be undermined for at least 1 cm. From my experience, flap undermining is not necessary in a virgin scalp to achieve a minimal scar.

Suturing Materials

Many methods of wound closure have been reported. It can be a one layer, two layers, deep plane fixation [9], or three layers closure. Some surgeons prefer to use staples [10] as they are quick to apply, but these are painful to remove. Haber [11] reported the use of dermabond to close the donor wound. I have no experience with this but believe that for a donor wound 1 cm wide or more the risk of wound dehiscence and a wide scar is high.

Nonabsorbable stitches are still widely used. They should be removed after 7–14 days. Nowadays many surgeons have turned to the use of absorbable stitches, saving the patients a trip to the clinic and the pain associated with removal of stitches.

James Arnold advocated the use of a tension clamp [12] to approximate the wound edge, leaving it in place for 10 min to reduce wound tension. The clamps are quick to apply, and on removal, wound closure becomes easier. I had been using this method in the past but was uncertain if wound tension can be reduced in just 10 min. Now I have changed to the use of retention stitches, which are less traumatic and can be left for 5–7 days, depending on the donor site width, without any problem. During this period the wound is constantly approximated, allowing the wound to heal with minimal tension. Good hemostasis can also be achieved.

Nordstrom et al. have introduced the Nordstrom suture [13] to enhance scalp reduction; it has potential use in repairing a wide donor scar but has never been released to the market for clinical use. Rassman [14] recently introduced the Quill suture in managing donor wound closure under tension. However, the result remains to be seen.

Retention Stitches (Figs. 3,4)

I have adopted a technique that seems to produce less of a scar (1–2 mm) when compared to my previous layers closure and deep plane fixation. I use a retention

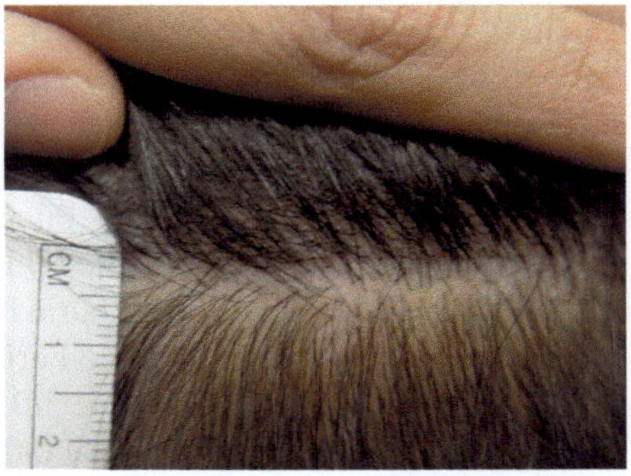

Fig. 3. Minimal donor scar

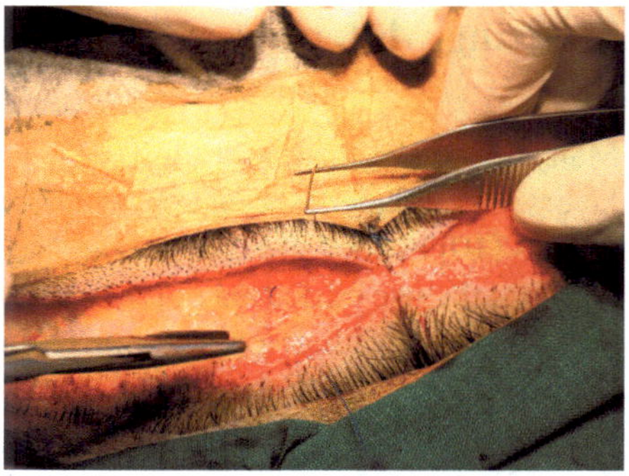

Fig. 4. Retention suture

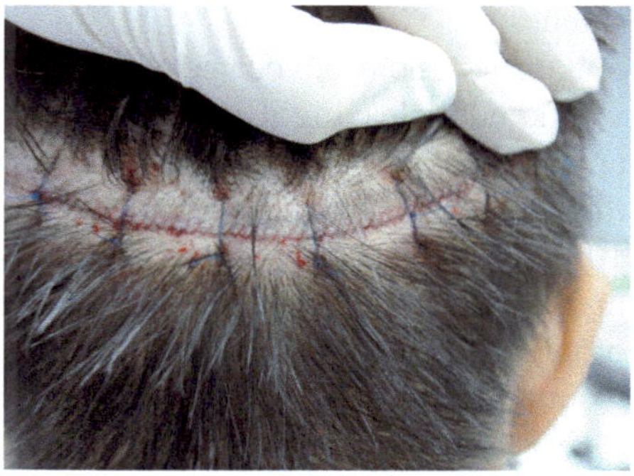

Fig. 5. Retention suture with 3/0 nylon

suture as my workhorse when there is bleeding or when the strip width exceeds 1 cm. A retention suture has been used in abdominal surgery for many decades [15–17]. It results in mechanical creep and creates biological creep if it stays longer. So far, no cross-hatching, stitch marks, or tissue necrosis has been encountered in more than 1000 cases.

First Session

If the strip is 1 cm or less, I close the wound as a single layer using absorbable stitches: 4/0 vicryl rapide (polyglactin 910) is my personal preference. Only a few patients have complained it takes too long for the stitches to dissolve. This material also causes less tissue reaction than monocryl [18], which I abandoned 5 years ago.

The needle takes a small bite on the skin edge down to the upper dermis, going over and over as a running suture. Pitchon advocated burying the knot on each end to reduce the pain [19]. I have tried this on many patients but did not observe any difference in pain between the buried and nonburied knot. I am also concerned about foreign-body reaction at the buried knot site.

For a strip 1–1.5 cm wide I use 3/0 nylon [20] as a retention suture, spacing at 1 in., followed by 4/0 vicryl rapide closure as described above.

For a strip 1.5–2 cm wide, I determine the width of the strip using Mayer-Paul's scalp elasticity scale [21]. Before suturing, I test the wound tension by approximating the skin edges with two skin hooks. If the scalp is very loose I do not undermine. The wound is closed as one layer with a retention suture followed by running vicryl as described. If the wound is tight I undermine upper and lower flaps until the skin edges can be approximated with minimal tension by the two skin hooks. The depth of the undermined flap on each side is then approximated by the retention suture every 2–3 cm depending on the tension. The stitches are removed in 5–7 days depending on the tension at the time of closure.

I stopped using layer closure because the suturing material as a foreign body may cause tissue reaction. In my experience this technique did not make the scar any smaller than retention sutures. Other surgeons might use one or two layers, absorbable or nonabsorbable sutures, or skin staples.

Subsequent Sessions

If the strip is 1 cm in width I use retention stitches without undermining.

For 1–2 cm, the flaps are undermined on both sides, passing over any nearby scars, until the skin edges are easily approximated by the pair of skin hooks. Retention stitches are then applied followed by vicryl rapide 4/0.

For the very tight scalp that cannot be closed I follow Beehner's recommendation [22]. The incision is packed with wet normal saline. Closure is reattempted at the end of the procedure when tumescent fluid is starting to wear off. If it is still not possible to close I would leave it open, packing with wet gauze to heal by secondary intention or skin grafting.

Other surgeons use a different approach to close the wound: two-layer closure with or without undermining, skin staples, or nonabsorbable sutures.

References

1. Hitzig G, Schwinmng J, Handler SL. Clinical application of infrared coagulator in hair transplantation. (Address reprint request to Gary Hitzig, 165 N. Village Ave, Ste. 125, Rochville Centre, NY 11570)
2. Warmuth IP, Massey RA Saintil M, et al (1998) Infrared coagulator in hair transplantation. Dermatol Surg 24:1079–1082 (32 refs)
3. Frechet P (2005) Donor harvesting with invisible scars. HT Forum Int 15(4)
4. Marzola M (2005) Trichophytic closure of the donor area. HT Forum Int 15(4)
5. Marzola M (2006) Single-scar harvesting technique. In: Haber R, Stough D (eds) Hair transplantation. Elsevier Saunders, Philadelphia, pp 83–85
6. Rose P (2005) Trichophytic donor closure. HT Forum Int 15(4)
7. Puig C (2008) Controlled trichophytic closure dissection with a ledge knife. Presented at annual scientific ISHRS meeting in Montreal, Canada

8. Kim DY (2008) Planning off inferior edge in Frechet & Rose trichophytic closure. Presented at annual scientific ISHRS meeting in Montreal, Canada
9. Gerald S (2002) Hair transplantation: management of the donor area. Dermatol Surg 28:136–142
10. Bernstein M (2008) Staples revisited. HT Forum Int 18:9
11. Haber R (2007) The use of octylcyanoacrylate-dermabond as a tissue adhesive for donor wound closure in hair transplantation. Hair Forum Int 33:966–971
12. Arnold J. Rapid intraoperative tissue expansion created by tension clamp. In: Haber RS, Stough DB (eds) Hair replacement: surgical and medical. Mosby, St. Louis, pp 259–266
13. Nordstrom RE, Greco M, Rapsio E, et al (2001) The Nordstrom suture to enhance scalp reduction. Plast Reconstruct Surg 107:583–585
14. Pak J, Rassman W, Gazoni P, et al (2008) Management of the occipital scalp tension wound in hair transplant surgery with the Quill suture. HT Forum Int 18:149
15. Wong SY, Kingsnorth AN (2002) Abdominal wound dehiscence and incisional hernia. Surgery (Oxf) 20:100–103
16. Parletic MM (2000) Use of external skin stretching device for wound closure in dogs and cats. J Am Vet Med Assoc 217:350–354
17 Moka G, Schonauer F, Blasi F (1999) Progressive skin extension: clinical and histological evaluation of a modified procedure using Kirshner wires. Br J Plast Surg 52:205–208
18. Lasinski J (2000) Monocryl suture in hair transplantation. HT Forum Int 10(3)
19. Pitchon M (2008) The good-night Closure. HT Forum Int 18:8
20. Brookside Associates (2001) Suture materials and techniques: use 3/0 nylon require good retention. Operational Medicine, Field Medical Service School Student handbook, p 99
21. Mayer M (2005) Scalp elasticity scale. HT Forum Int 15(4)
22. Beehner M (2000) A proposal for selective delayed closure of the donor area. HT Forum Int 10(3)

Donor Strip Removal and Wound Closure in Super Mega-Session: My Personal Technique

J. Wong

Donor strip removal is covered elsewhere in this book, so I just want to add a few pointers pertaining to wide strip excision. Once again unless the patient has a very loose scalp, almost everyone benefits from scalp stretching exercises, and this is especially true with subsequent surgeries where the scalp gets progressively tighter with each surgery. Even with experience at judging scalp laxity we will occasionally take too much and have difficulty closing despite undermining. If that happens it is sometimes best to leave a small gap and use postoperative antibiotic ointment to keep the area free from infection. Check the wound every few days until healing occurs, and the resulting wider scar can be revised at a later date if necessary. If there is any doubt regarding the scalp laxity, it is best to be conservative and not go so wide because 1 to 2 mm of additional width can greatly increase the closure tension. Drs. Mayer and Rassman both have laxity scales to measure donor laxity but these are only a guide. To avoid undue tension and still take out the maximum width, Dr. Mucie of Brazil has a harvesting technique that is probably fail safe and should work every time. She starts by making the inferior cut and then undermines the bottom of the strip. Vertical cuts are then made in the donor tissue and skin hooks are used to overlap the skin edges to determine the width that can be removed, very similar to what was done in the past for scalp reductions.

Currently I use Wong's three-finger wiggle test to determine strip width. Once the width of the strip is marked out I place the right thumb on the top line of the strip and the right index finger on the bottom line. The left index finger is placed over the center of the strip just above skin surface and held suspended with no movement. When the right thumb pulls the skin downward the top line should slide at least to the middle of the stationary left index finger. When the skin is pulled up by the right index finger the bottom line should slide at least up to the middle of the left index finger. The donor width can be adjusted depending on the ease and the amount of skin movement. This method is very reliable if we are not overly aggressive. Working on the edge trying to pull out as much hair as possible is a totally different game. Here, if we overshoot even by 2 mm, closure tension can increase from moderate to extreme.

D. Pathomvanich and K. Imagawa (eds.), *Hair Restoration Surgery in Asians*
DOI 10.1007/978-4-431-99659-0_24, © Springer 2010

Wound Closure

For widths up to 10 mm I use only skin staples; for anything wider than 10 mm I close with two layers. For the deep layer I use interrupted 4–0 vicryl spaced 0.5 to 1 in. apart, depending on how easily the edges come together. With tight closures I space the sutures a little closer together, cut the suture close to the knot, leaving as little suture material in the wound as possible. The deep suture helps to ease the tension on the skin layer and patients are more comfortable postoperatively. The suture needs to bite galea; the subcutaneous tissue is simply not strong enough. Try to keep the galeal bite small and try to avoid catching deep nerves and vessels. If the closure is very tight, instruct the patient to push his chin away from his chest and relax his neck muscles as this will ease skin tension, making the closure easier.

The skin surface is closed with staples (3 M), and the majority of our donors are closed under mild to moderate tension; staples are far superior to sutures when tension is involved. We have been fortunate in that so far we have not seen any vascular necrosis in the donor area.

Follicular Unit Extraction in the Asian Population

B. Ng

In 1988, Masumi Inaba in Japan introduced the use of a 1-mm punch for extracting individual follicular units. In 2002, Rassman refined the procedure and named it follicular unit extraction (FUE) or the FOX procedure (follicular unit extraction). FUE serves as an alternative to the use of a strip in donor harvesting [1]. FUE attracts the attention of those who desire hair transplantation but are turned off by a linear donor scar.

Being a blind technique, the number of grafts is limited by a high transection rate. Over the years many different FUE techniques have evolved to overcome this problem [2–4]. A five-step personal approach is described in the first part of this chapter.

The real problem of FUE, however, is the depletion of donor grafts for future sessions. The second part outlines the considerations when offering a FUE megasession to those Asian subgroups who have low hair density and a low hair-to-graft ratio (e.g., Chinese, Japanese, Thai) [5,6].

Part I: Personal FUE Technique

Instruments

When using the FUE round punch, the 0.75- to 0.8-mm size should be reserved for one-hair FU. The 1.0-mm size can be used for most two- and three-hair grafts. The larger 1.2-mm punch, with potential to leave a scar and transect adjacent follicles, should be avoided [1].

The "Vari-handle" is recommended as punch holder for three reasons:

1. A blocked punch will create buried grafts. Tissue debris can be irrigated out through the slot of the handle.
2. Depth control of the punch can be set.
3. The weight and length of the handle helps to control the tip on scoring.

D. Pathomvanich and K. Imagawa (eds.), *Hair Restoration Surgery in Asians*
DOI 10.1007/978-4-431-99659-0_25, © Springer 2010

A curved forceps provides a larger contact area for a better grip of the graft. A second pair of straight forceps is needed for difficult extraction.

Surgical loupes provide good visualization. Magnification higher than 2× may cause more eyestrain.

Moist dressing material instead of a gloved finger should be used to collect extracted grafts (see Fig. 4) before transferring to a Petri dish with cool saline [7].

Preoperative Preparation

Gray or white hair should be colored before surgery. The FOX test has been advocated for patient selection, especially for a mega-session [8]. In real practice, it is rather time consuming and unreliable. What initially appears to be difficult may turn out to be an easy extraction after the surgeon adapts the technique to cater for the angle and direction of the follicles. The entire donor site should be trimmed leaving behind 0.3–0.5 cm of hair above the skin to guide the punch. Those reluctant to shave must have kept the hair long enough to cover one or two trimmed windows.

Scalp laxity should be assessed [9]. A very tight scalp alerts the possibility of underlying idiopathic tissue fibrosis, which necessitates deeper scoring.

Positions

The patient's comfort must be ensured as FUE takes many hours. The patient should lie in a prone position with the surgeon sitting either by the side or at the end of the table.

Inspect the hair at the occiput and parietal areas. The surgeon should start at an easy area to gain confidence.

The patient's neck should be flexed when harvesting the inferior donor area. Here the hair usually exits at a flat angle and stretching the scalp helps to erect the follicles.

Marking the FUE Donor Area

The "safe margins" of the donor area should be marked to avoid picking up non-permanent hair. There is no fixed rule in defining the safe donor areas. However, Unger and Alt's recommendations may be used as a guideline [10].

Looking for grafts at the end of procedure is frustrating. One practical tip is to divide the marked donor area into small blocks of similar sizes.

N = the planned number of grafts
n = the number of blocks
N/n = the number of grafts to be harvested per block

If this number cannot be obtained in a defined block, the surgeon should prepare to expand the donor area or to accept lesser grafts.

Local Anesthesia and Tumescence

The local anesthetic of personal choice should be injected below and along the inferior border.

Tumescence fluid should not be injected as routine. The ease of extraction must first be tested with and without tumescence. It should be injected intradermally, a small area at a time, and away from "holes" to avoid spilling.

Graft Selection

From personal experience, a random approach may obtain more multi-FU grafts than an orderly approach in extraction.

All healthy-looking multi-FUs within a block should first be randomly extracted. On the second round, one-hair grafts are extracted.

One rule must be followed: those grafts next to an empty hole should be spared.

The Five-Step Approach

Straighforward FUE requires only two steps: scoring and extraction [11]. When extraction is difficult with high transection, a five-step approach is necessary.

Step 1: Indentation

The sharp tip of the punch may slip and transect the underside of the follicle. The punch should be secured on the skin surface before scoring.

After containing the hairs of a FU, the punch is positioned vertically on the skin surface. It is then pushed downward to create an indentation on the skin, which in return embraces the punch (Fig. 1).

Step 2: Sharp Scoring

The angle of the punch is changed to align with the hair.

The handle is rotated to-and-fro with the thumb, index, and middle fingers to advance the punch.

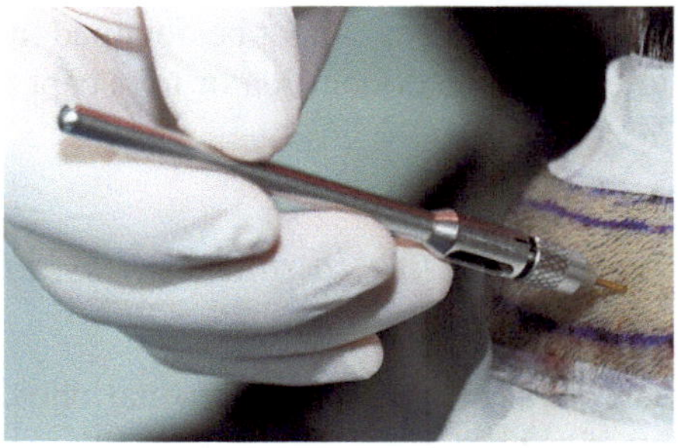

Fig. 1. Indentation

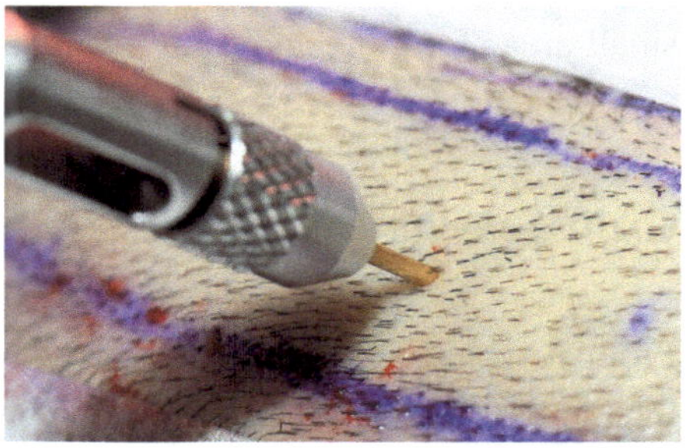

Fig. 2. Scoring

Scoring should stop when tissue resistance is felt, which usually occurs on cutting the arector pili at the isthmus [12]. Beyond this point, the tissue will suddenly give way so that the punch may drop too deep and transect the roots (Fig. 2).

Step 3: Test Extraction

Single-Forceps Technique

One common problem encountered in extraction is "de-capping:" by just grasping a small amount of tissue the skin only is removed without the follicle.

The tips of the curved forceps are opened, placed around the dissected follicle, and pressed down upon the surrounding skin. The exposed upper dermis of the popped-up follicle is then grasped firmly by the same forceps.

The graft is "pushed" rather than "pulled" out by pronating the wrist (Fig. 3).

Double-Forceps Technique

If de-capping still occurs, the follicle is first held and lifted by the curved forceps as described. A second pair of straight forceps is positioned below the curved forceps to grasp lower and extract the graft. This step can be performed by an assistant.

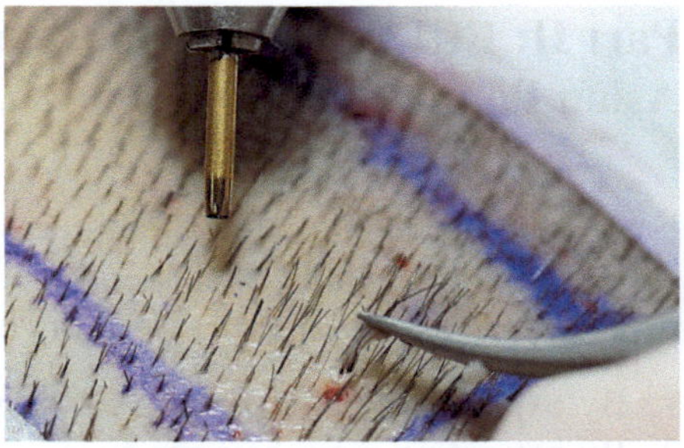

Fig. 3. Extraction

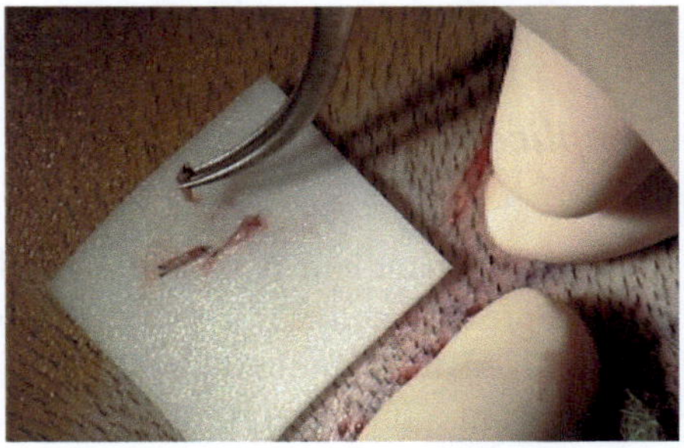

Fig. 4. Placing the grafts on a wet dressing material

Any de-capped graft should be left behind. The struggle to remove it may create a buried graft.

There is a learning curve for each case. The first 15 to 30 min should be spent patiently testing the proper angle, direction, and depth of the punch. Successful extraction requires no further action, but if the graft fails to come out, the next two steps become necessary.

Steps 4 and 5: Deep Dissection and Re-Extraction

Three different tools can be used to free the follicle from any deep tethering before re-extraction:

1. Using Dr. Harris' dull punch [4,13]
2. Using a sharp needle tip as recommended by Dr. Rassman [11]
3. Using the same punch to cut deeper but with a lesser force and speed

These two steps are repeated until the graft is removed.

Postoperative Care of the Donor Site

The usual postop protocol applies. Dressing is only needed in perfuse oozing. A moisturizing ointment or mild topical steroid-antibiotic preparation may be used to relieve dryness and itchiness.

Part II: FUE Mega-Session: Special Considerations in Asian Populations

For Asian populations, the difficulties in FUE usually arise from a discrepancy between high demand [14–17] and low supply of donor hair [5,6]. There are two ways to increase the number of grafts but at a higher risk for complications:

1. By expanding the harvesting area into unsafe zones
2. By extracting more hair per square centimeter.

Complications

1. Nonpermanent hair is picked up by harvesting a nonsafe area.
2. FUE prevents a linear scar but it is not a scarless technique [1]. As a larger area is utilized, the cumulative scarring of open wounds is in fact significantly greater than from a linear incision.
3. Empty spots, "snail tracks," and mottling occur when adjacent follicles are extracted (Figs. 5, 6). These markings are more visible in Asians with high hair–scalp color contrast.
4. Thinning occurs as a result of the selective extraction of two- to three-hair FUs in a low-density donor area [18]. Any underlying scars or mottling becomes more obvious.
5. Depletion of donor density leading to a wider scar if strip is required for subsequent sessions.

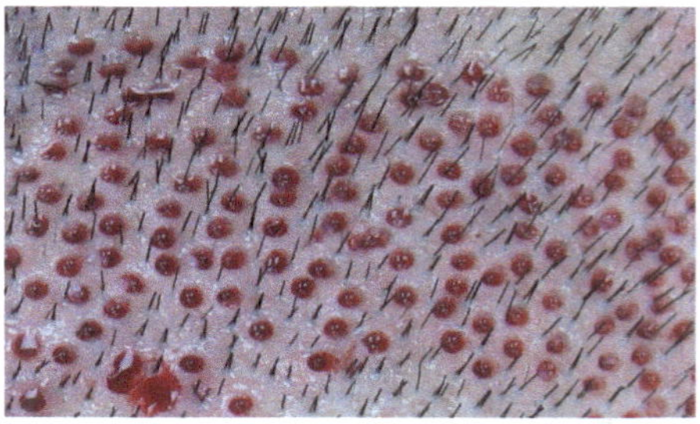

Fig. 5. Extractions too close to each other

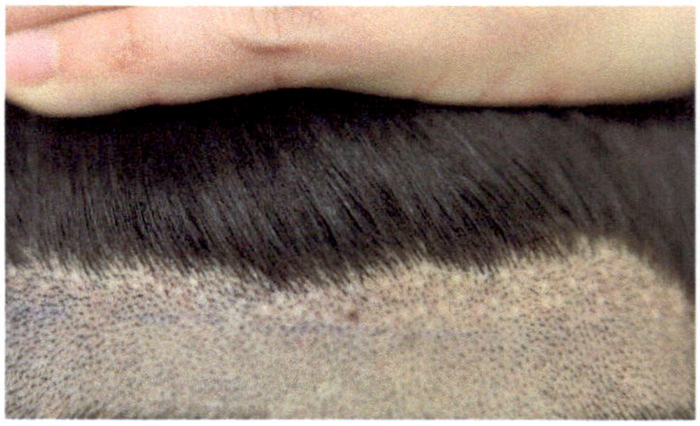

Fig. 6. Follicular unit extraction (FUE) can leave patchy scars

Advantages of FUE

1. One doctor and one or two assistants can run a center.
2. The procedure is less traumatic, and less surgical experience is required.
3. Graft preparation is minimal, requiring less equipment.
4. Less postoperative discomfort for the patient, with no need to remove sutures.
5. Minimal scarring if only a limited number of grafts is harvested.

Indications for FUE

1. Removal of unwanted grafts.
2. Selective extraction of single-hair FUs for eyebrow or eyelash transplant.
3. When only a small number of grafts is required and further strip excision is not anticipated.
4. When patients do not accept a linear donor scar.

Poor Candidates for FUE

1. The patient does not care about the donor scar.
2. A future strip is anticipated to complete the job; for example, the very young patient with early class III.
3. The patient has a limited budget but requires the maximum in one session.

References

1. Gökrem S, Baser NT, Aslan G (2008) Follicular unit extraction in hair transplantation: personal experience. Ann Plast Surg 60:127–133
2. Lorenzo J (2007) FUE: tools vs. skill. Abstract, ISHRS 15th annual scientific meeting, Las Vegas, NV
3. Rassman W, Harris J, Bernstein R (2006) Follicular unit extraction. In: Haber R, Stough D (eds) Hair transplantation. Elsevier Saunders, Philadelphia, pp 133–142
4. Harris JA (2006) New methodology and instrumentation for follicular unit extraction: lower follicle transection rates and expanded patient candidacy. Dermatol Surg 32:56–61; discussion 61–62. Comment in Dermatol Surg 2006;32(4):599
5. Pathomvanich D (2002) A random study of Asian male androgenic alopecia in Bangkok, Thailand. Dermatol Surg 28:804–807
6. Tsai RY, Lee SH, Chan HL (2002) The distribution of follicular units in the Chinese scalp: implications for reconstruction of natural-appearing hairlines in Orientals. Dermatol Surg 28:500–503
7. Cooley J (2006) Achieving optimal growth. In: Haber R, Stough D (eds) Hair transplantation. Elsevier Saunders, Philadelphia, pp 111–116

8. Bernstein R, Rassman W, Anderson K (2004) FUE megasessions: evolution of a technique. HT Forum Int 14:97–99
9. Mayer M (2005) Scalp elasticity scale. HT Forum Int 15(4)
10. Unger W, Cole J (2004) The donor area. In: Unger WP, Shapiro R (eds) Hair transplantation, 4th edn. Dekker, New York, pp 301–304
11. Rassman W, Harris J, Bernstein R (2006) Follicular unit extraction. In: Haber RS, Stough D (eds) Hair transplantation. Elsevier Saunders, Philadelphia, pp 133–142
12. Poblet E, Ortega F, Jimenez F (2002) The arrector pili muscle and the follicular unit of the scalp: a microscopic anatomy study. Dermatol Surg 28:800–903
13. Harris J (2007) FUE: potential pitfalls, problems, and remedies. Abstract, ISHRS 15th annual scientific meeting, Las Vegas, NV
14. Pathomvanich D (2006) Hair transplant in Asian. In: Haber RS, Stough D (eds) Hair transplantation. Elsevier Saunders, Philadelphia pp 149–156
15. Bernstein RM, Rassman WR (1997) The aesthetics of follicular transplantation. Dermatol Surg 23:785–99
16. Le TT, Farkas LG, Ngim RC, et al (2002) Proportionality in Asian and North American Caucasian faces using neoclassical facial canons as criteria. Aesthetic Plast Surg 26:64–69
17. Beehner M (1997) A frontal forelock/central density framework for hair transplantation. Dermatol Surg 23:807–815
18. Ruifernandez JF (1999) Distribution of human hair in follicular units. A mathematical model of estimating the donor size in follicular unit transplantation. Dermatol Surg 25:294–298

Part VIII
Graft Preparation: Personal Techniques

Slivering and Graft Cutting

K. Amonpattana, R. Palakurthi, P. Thienthaworn, and S. Manochai

Graft preparation is an important part of hair transplant surgery, requiring a combination of skill and experience. Because Dr. Pathomvanich's refined open technique demands more time to accomplish this, we usually remove the first 5 to 7 cm of the strip and send it to the assistants for prompt slivering without any delay. The remaining strip is subsequently dissected into pieces to keep up with the speed of the slivering assistants. This size caters to our specially designed slivering chamber.

Slivering

The strip is pinned, using two to four 23 G needles, onto a silicon block in one of the chambers filled with cool saline; this is to ensure the dermal papilla is well hydrated at all times. The slivering is done either with a 3× magnifying loupe or under a 10× video image with an external cool light (Fig. 1). We do not use a microscope for slivering as the focus cannot be maintained on handling a thick piece of tissue.

A skin hook is applied to the proximal free end of the strip, held by the non-dominant hand, with steady lateral traction to open up the sliver. The dominant hand exercises a no. 15 blade to first score along the skin surface with the bevel, followed by downstroke cutting with its sharp tip.

We prefer to sliver along the longer side of the strip. We found that in most cases the follicles align in rows along the length of the strip, leaving some space in between for transection-free slivering. Also, it is always more difficult to open up a sliver, and this is encountered less often by cutting a longer piece. Moreover, tension can be easily maintained in opening up the follicles. Nevertheless, as it takes longer to dissect one sliver when compared to cutting across, we have designed our chamber to ensure that the strip is always immersed in saline solution.

One or two rows of the follicular units can be included in one sliver. We prefer two rows as this piece is neither too thick nor too thin. Too thin a slivered piece increases the chance of traumatizing the hair bulbs. Too thick a slivered piece

D. Pathomvanich and K. Imagawa (eds.), *Hair Restoration Surgery in Asians*
DOI 10.1007/978-4-431-99659-0_26,

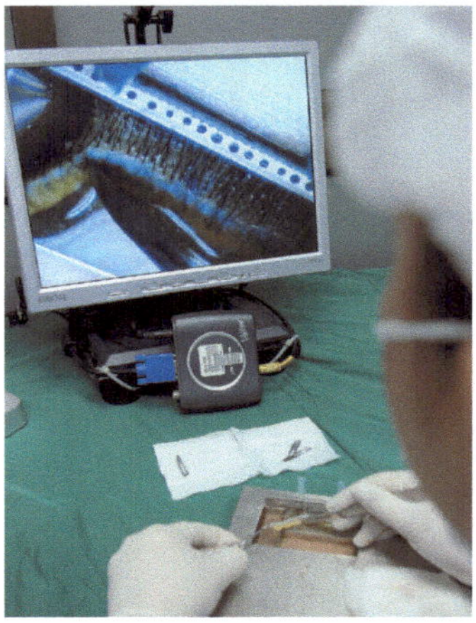

Fig. 1. Slivering in our slivering chamber under video image

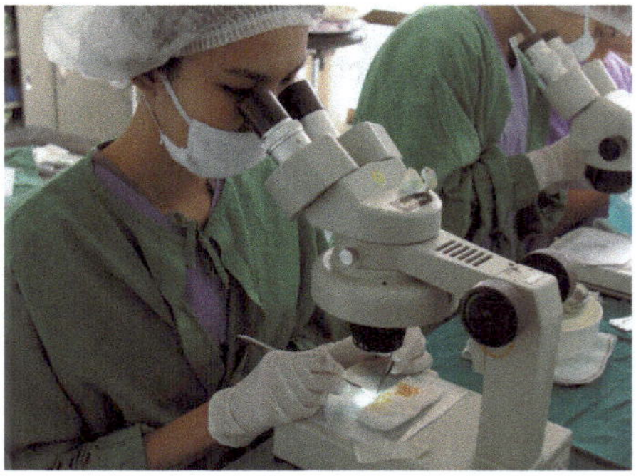

Fig. 2. Graft cutting under microscopes

would lose the benefit of backlighting in microscopic graft dissection. From our experience, this technique results in very minimal follicular transection.

Graft Cutting

We routinely use a stereoscopic microscope with 10× magnification (Fig. 2). A piece of plastic sheet (polyvinyl chloride, PVC) is used as a cutting sheet as this has several advantages:

- It allows transillumination of the backlight
- Its surface can be roughened to prevent graft sliding
- It is not so hard as to dull the blade rapidly
- It is not so soft that pieces can be chipped off as potential foreign bodies
- It does not draw away moisture from the grafts

We use no. 10 Swann-Morton scalpel blades for cutting. The blades are changed when they get dull to avoid unnecessary transection. For tough skin we prefer to

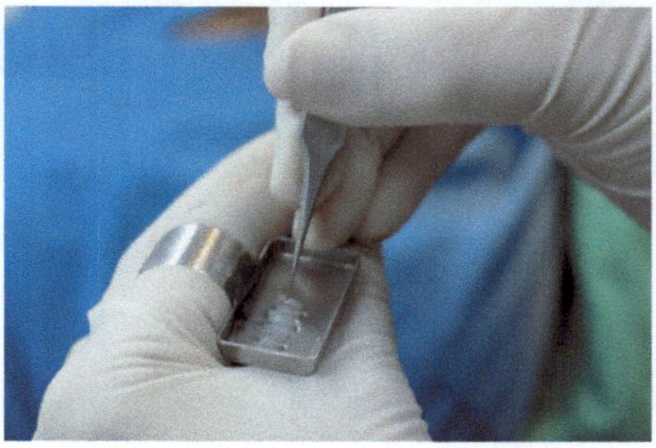

Fig. 3. The "ring" for holding grafts

use a Personna Plus Blade as it is the sharpest blade available on the market. Unfortunately, this blade is not available worldwide.

The subcutaneous fat in the slivers is usually first trimmed away to leave 1 mm below the follicles. A small amount of fat can hold the roots together for easy insertion. Also, grasping the fat instead of the papilla will minimize graft damage during insertion.

Care must be taken in preparing white hair grafts as their "invisible" papillae are always longer than those of the pigmented ones and can easily be cut away on fat trimming. Some surgeons recommended turning off all lights except the backlight to minimize distraction.

We also prefer to leave a small rim of epithelium around the hair shaft as a yardstick during insertion to prevent tenting and pitting. The grafts are then rinsed with chilled saline to wash away any unwanted particles before being separated into one-hair, two-hair, and three-hair follicular units.

We use chilled normal saline as stock solution as it is easily available at low cost. Some surgeons prefer to keep the grafts in Hypothermosol (from Biolife Solution), Moser Machte media, or Ringer's lactate solution, which are reported to be more "physiological" in containing nutrients and antioxidant [1,3] in an optimal pH.

Over the past few years platelet-rich plasma (PRP) was introduced in hair transplantation and documented to enhance the growth of the transplanted hair [2]. This may be the stock solution of the future if the preparation can be simplified.

The surgeon is informed of the number of counted grafts to plan the incisions. We have designed a graft-holding ring made of lightweight stainless steel that fits comfortably to the finger for ergonomic graft insertion (Fig. 3).

An Alternative Way of Graft Cutting

J.-C. Kim

The excised strip is placed on a block of birchwood and sectioned into smaller segments using a no. 20 scalpel blade, with careful positioning of the blade between and at the same angle as the visible hair follicles (Fig. 4). With the same blade, each segment is then cut again into follicular units. Grafts are closely trimmed to eliminate all unneeded dermis and subcutaneous tissue, thereby providing very clean and neatly trimmed grafts. Clean and closely trimmed grafts allow for implantation in a greater density than grafts that are allowed to carry with them all surrounding dermis.

The grafts should be placed in a Petri dish with gauze or Telfa pads that has been at least half-filled with cold saline. Survival of preserved hair grafts is better at 4°C than at room temperature. Storage of prepared grafts on gauze or Telfa pads (in air–fluid interface) can increase the integrity of hair grafts as compared with floating storage (submerged preservation) (Fig. 5). If the grafts are immersed, the grafts absorb excess solution, which causes greater difficulty during placement into the needle of the implanter.

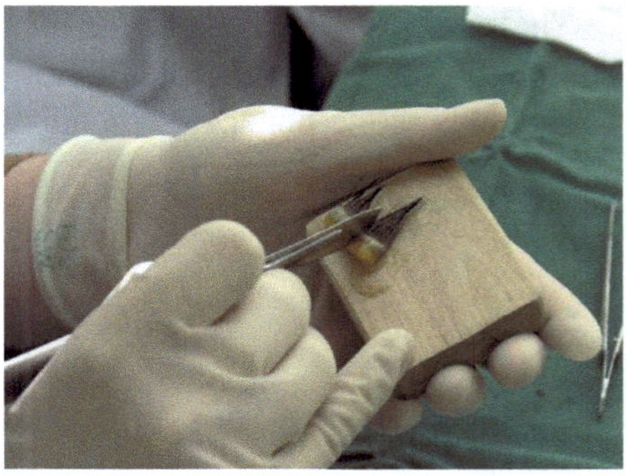

Fig. 4. Graft cutting on a wood block

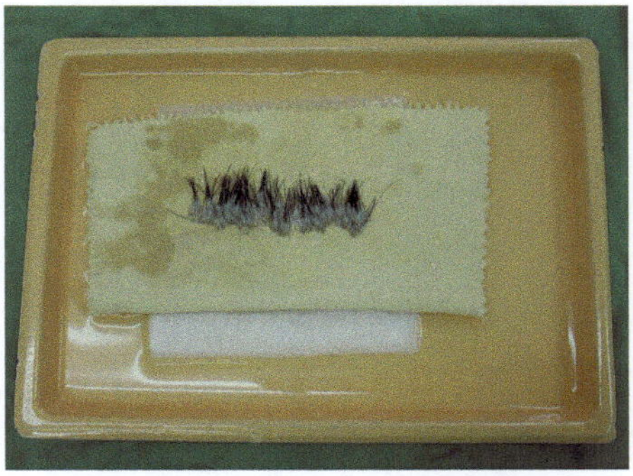

Fig. 5. Storage of grafts to improve air–fluid interface

References

1. Greco J, Brandt RJ (2005) Maximizing the use of autologous platelet rich plasma in hair transplantation surgery. Internet website posting, Dec 3, 2008, www.regrowhair.com
2. Uebel CO (2004) Graft survival and platelet rich plasma. Presented at the annual scientific meeting of the American Society of Plastic Surgeons in Philadelphia, PA, Oct 9–13
3. Walter P (2004) Graft preparation. In: Unger WP, Shapiro R (eds) Hair transplantation, 4th edn. Dekker, New York, 349–380
4. Bouhanna P, Dardour JC (1996) Hair replacement surgery textbook and atlas. Springer, New York, pp 70–102
5. Barrera A (2002) Hair transplantation: the art of micrograft and minigraft. Quality Medical, St. Louis, MO, pp 47–120

Graft Dissection in Super Mega-Session: My Personal Technique

J. Wong

I will restrict my comments on graft dissections not to the mechanics of how to dissect grafts but to staff utilization for these large sessions. Our full surgical team consists of ten surgical assistants, and when everyone is present we are slightly overstaffed. For cost efficiency, 4000 to 4500 grafts can be done comfortably with six or seven experienced staff members, but if more than one member is off work for reasons of holiday or illness, then it can be quite stressful to work understaffed. If those away are key members then it becomes very difficult, if not impossible, to do large sessions. It is much more comfortable to have the extra help and not have to worry about shortages. With the extra help, the inserters (key members) do not have to worry about graft dissections and can concentrate on placing grafts. The majority of our staff can sliver, dissect and place grafts, and the goal is to eventually have everyone proficient at doing all three jobs.

For ease of handling and to work efficiently, the strip is taken out in three sections. The first section is removed as the majority of the staff members arrive and graft dissection starts while donor removal continues. Initially, we have nine assistants dissecting grafts while one assists with the strip removal. By the time the remaining donor strip is removed and the recipient sites made, there are more than sufficient grafts to keep up to three inserters busy. The grafts are stored on wet gauze using Plasmalyte solution and are chilled. Every cutter has their own ice tray to keep both the slivers and grafts chilled. Because the cutting is always quicker than graft insertion, a cover is placed over the graft dishes to prevent dehydration while they sit waiting to be used.

Microscopic dissection enables the experienced technician to trim grafts with greater accuracy and precision. Many used to argue that loupe dissection produces grafts of similar quality, but in our experience, once the staff members became efficient with the microscopes, it was impossible to go back to loupe magnifiers. The microscope's improved visibility allow more excess skin and fat to be trimmed away, producing slim, accurately trimmed grafts that will fit into smaller slits. In addition to improving graft quality, microscopic slivering (popularized by David Seager) reduced graft wastage. As a result, we not only have better grafts but now we have more grafts (sometime as much as 30% more) from the same size of donor strip.

D. Pathomvanich and K. Imagawa (eds.), *Hair Restoration Surgery in Asians*
DOI 10.1007/978-4-431-99659-0_27, © Springer 2010

Quality control to track both quality and wastage is an ongoing issue and requires the surgeon to spend that extra 20 to 30 min looking over the assistant's shoulder. I have tried to assign this "quality control" job to a staff member but have not been successful. Dr. Tony Rouston of Brazil may have the answer to this problem. He has one of his assistants checking everyone's grafts and correcting any grafts that are less than perfect. This system works extremely well as the quality of his team's grafts is excellent.

Part IX
Recipient Site Preparation and Insertion

Dense Packing

J. Wong

It has long been recognized that density is largely dependent upon blade size: a smaller blade results in more slits in any given area. Dense packing is defined as placing grafts at 28 or more follicular units (FU)/cm^2. As a consequence of stereoscopic dissection the physical size of grafts has gradually decreased. These smaller grafts require smaller recipient slits, and today it is possible, in people with smaller and shorter follicles, to densely pack up to 45/cm^2 two-hair FUs (sometimes more) and still obtain consistent growth. For example a 0.85-mm blade set at up to 4.5 mm deep is generally safe at 45/cm^2. Two-hair FUs in Asians usually require a 0.95-mm blade set at a depth of 5 mm. Even with such a slight increase in blade size and dense packing at 45/cm^2 may reduce growth in some individuals. Reasonable starting densities for most surgeons are at around 25 to 28 FU/cm^2, and these numbers may be slowly increased if there are no growth issues. For beginners, or those with new surgical teams, I would suggest that you start with whatever the team is comfortable with and do not dense pack until the skill level improves. There are wide variations in the manual skills of both surgeon and teams, so that what is safe for one group may be unsafe for another.

Even in healthy patients without risk factors, the tolerance for dense packing will vary considerably. What may work for the first 30 patients may not work for the 31st, and it takes but a handful of bad results to ruin a reputation. Use caution and space the grafts a little further apart when the blade depth reaches 5 mm. Occasionally we see follicles that are greater than 5 mm in length, but in these cases there is usually no need to cut deeper than 5 mm. The longer grafts will generally seat quite well in a shorter slit, but always check with a few test slits first to make sure that is the case and increase the depth slightly if required.

Before cutting slits, it is extremely important to create tumescence of the skin. We use a mixture of 100 ml saline + 0.4 ml 1 : 1000 adrenalin + 10 ml 2% xylocaine. Creating tumescence in the subcutaneous space will increase the separation between the skin surface and the deep vessels and at the same time increase skin turgor; this will reduce damage to the deep vessels as we cut slits. I believe this step is vital before cutting slits and should be done every time. It may lessen the incidence of serious complications, such as vascular necrosis.

Some hair transplant surgeons are using steroid in either oral or intramuscular form after surgery to prevent facial swelling. More commonly, the steroid is added to the tumescence fluid in different strengths. I have been using triamcinolone

D. Pathomvanich and K. Imagawa (eds.), *Hair Restoration Surgery in Asians*
DOI 10.1007/978-4-431-99659-0_28, © Springer 2010

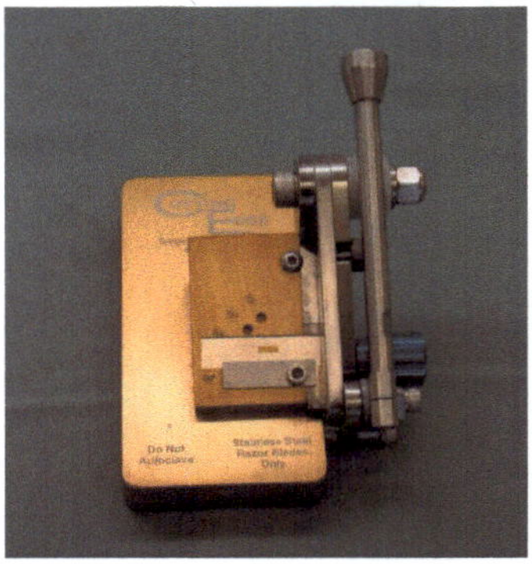

Fig. 1. Cutter designed to cut Personna single-edge prep blades

20 mg in 120 normal saline and found significant reduction in facial edema. Later I cut down to 10 mg but did not see such improvement. Because I am doing dense packing and mega-sessions I am not quite sure about the negative impact of steroid on hair growth. Consequently, I have stopped its use for a while and may reconsider its use in the future.

Regardless of the cutting instrument used to make the slits, the goal is to minimize skin damage as much as possible. Again, we do this by using the correct blade for graft size, controlling the blade depth, and tumescing the region before cutting sites. Also, the cutting instrument needs to be sharp. If we use a dull blade, needle, or punch, there will be increased skin damage resulting in poor growth or worse. At one time there were few commercially available blades for making recipient sites and the ones that were available were far too big for the new grafts. Dr. Hasson and I assisted Roy Ratson of Cutting Edge Surgical to develop a blade cutter to cut recipient blades from Personna prep blades (Fig. 1).

The cutter can generate "custom-cut" razor-sharp blades of any size from 0.5 to 4.0 mm or larger. The combination of exact size and depth minimizes skin damage, allowing mega-sessions to be done safely. This custom-cut blade should be so sharp that it will cut with virtually no resistance even through scar tissue. When surgeries are done with precision and attention to detail, problems such as visible scaring, pitting of grafts, and ridging of the hairline are now rarely seen.

Dense packing is an ongoing process of continuous refinement, and the numbers presented are only general guidelines. How close any surgical team can pack is dependent on the size and quality of the grafts, the care given to the handling and storage of grafts, the skill of the inserters, etc. As the team's overall skill improves, the density of graft planting may be slowly increased, providing there are no concerns about subsequent poor growth of the grafts. The ultimate density that is achievable differs from team to team. Just because one surgical team can successfully transplant at 50 to 60 FU/cm^2 does not mean that everyone else can. One should increase the numbers only if there are no growth problems with your current density. No one other than yourself can determine what the current safe limits are for your team or ultimately how close your team can pack. Detailed records need to be kept regarding blade size, spacing, and depth so that on follow-up visits we can track what works and what needs adjusting.

Premade Incisions: When and Where to Begin

J. Wong

A few years back we were routinely doing 6000+ graft cases. The excessive work and the long hours of these large cases began to cause shoulder, wrist, and back problems for the inserting staff. We still do the occasional 6000-graft case but these are not done routinely. Most of the time we try to limit the size of the surgeries to a maximum of 5500 grafts. As the first surgery is usually the largest session, it is a good idea to ease the workload and do only relatively easy areas: this is that vast area on the top of the head extending from the hairline back to the crown swirl. Because the hair in this area mostly faces the same direction and the area is large enough to allow two (occasionally three) inserters to work simultaneously, 4000 to 5000 grafts can usually be finished in 8 to 10 h. Crown swirls and temple restorations, which are more time consuming, are usually reserved for the second surgery when the session is much smaller. Asian hair, because of decreased density and laxity, will generally yield 3000 to 4000 grafts on average, and 4500 grafts are usually the maximum that is obtainable. Thus, we seldom have to worry about 6000-graft days.

With mega-sessions we need to work as efficiently as possible as 10 to 15 min added here or there will greatly prolong the case. Once the donor strip is out and while the doctor is numbing the recipient area, one of the assistants will load and set up the blade handles.

We have six blade handles for every case, and because blades must be changed at the first sign of dullness, having several handles will reduce downtime. We begin by cutting slits at the frontal one-third beginning at the lower margin; slits are cut in rows working forward. The frontal one-third needs to look as natural as possible regardless of how the patient wears his or her hair; therefore, I like to use all single- and double-hair grafts in this area. At the start 1200 to 1400 double-hair slits will be cut, leaving a 1.0- to 1.5-cm zone at the hairline for the single-hair grafts; this is usually enough room to pack in 700 to 800 singles at the hairline. Due to its dark color and coarseness, Asian hair requires at least 500 to 700 singles to produce a soft hairline, and with a mega-session these numbers are easily generated. Until we gain more experience as to how much space to leave for the single follicles, we may choose to cut single slits at the hairline first and follow with the doubles directly behind. However, if the doubles are cut first, the single blade, because of

D. Pathomvanich and K. Imagawa (eds.), *Hair Restoration Surgery in Asians*
DOI 10.1007/978-4-431-99659-0_29, © Springer 2010

its smaller size, does a better job filling any small gaps between the double and single slits.

Once the two-hair sites are nearly done the assistant will load four or five handles with blades (0.65–0.7 mm) for the single grafts. Cutting 800 single and 1200 double sites is usually sufficient for two inserters to work. However, if the plan is to use three inserters then I will cut another 500 large slits toward the crown to allow room for a third inserter (Figs. 1–3).

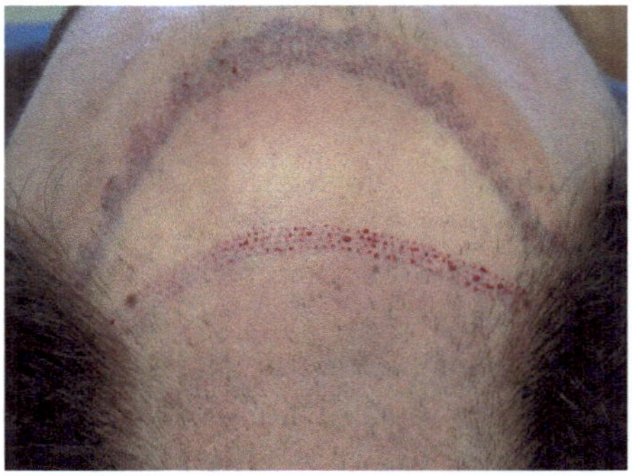

Fig 1. Singles cut first and bottom four rows of doubles cut

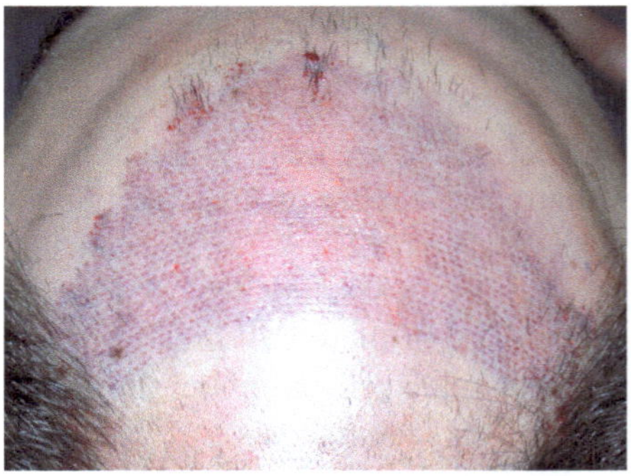

Fig 2. Frontal area slits cut

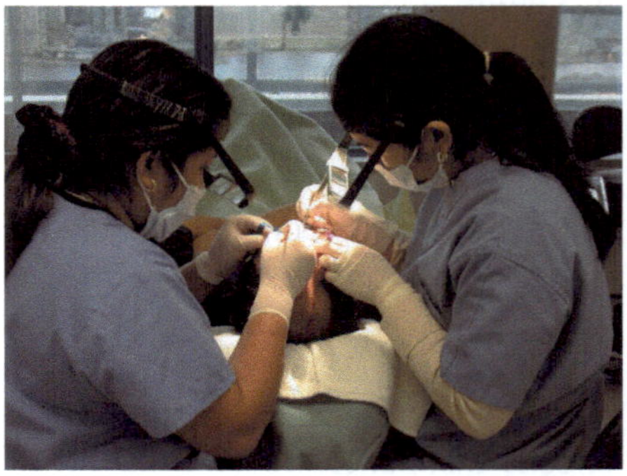

Fig 3. Two people plantingsd

If two inserters are used, we wait until after the double slits are mostly filled before making any more slits to minimize blood ooze from the sites. Directly behind the doubles we place the three- to four-hair FUs, and these will range from 400 to 900 grafts depending on the individual. The size of these larger FUs may vary requiring different sized blades. Most of the time we will use a 1.2-mm blade, spacing the slits at 20 to 25 FU/cm^2.

By placing the larger grafts further back in the mid-scalp there often are some fine residual hairs remaining, and these will soften and blend in the larger grafts. Also, the mid-scalp is the least visible area, making it an ideal site for these larger grafts. The remaining two-hair grafts are placed posterior to the larger grafts toward the crown region. The crown area is highly visible and should be done with smaller grafts. If larger grafts are used in the crown area, they should be placed toward the periphery, preferable in the thinning hair margin where the thin residual hair can help to soften and blend these larger grafts. Do not place large grafts near the center of the swirl. In most cases there may be 100 to 200 one-hair grafts left at the end of the day, and these can be used to soften the posterior hairline, or they may be used to "stick-and-place" any missed areas.

Patients will often request that we spread the remaining grafts over the entire crown area for a thinning look rather than stopping with a posterior hairline. This is not a good idea because transplanted hairs will not look good if spaced too far apart. It is far better to create a soft hairline in the back and transplant the crown later. Always soften the back line as some patient may not come back for further crown work.

Why Lateral Slits?

J. Wong

Back in the days of mini-/micro-grafting when larger grafts containing five to eight hairs were placed in sagittal slits, the transplanted hair exited the skin in a perpendicular fashion, creating a very unnatural look. By turning the blade 90°, pointing the handle in the direction of hair flow, and tilting the handle to match the exit angle of the residual hairs, the slit will sandwich the graft and hold it at the precut slit angle. Laterally directed slits provide an effective means to control the transplanted hair's exit angle as it emerges from the skin. When transplanted hair matches the existing hair's exit angle, a much more natural look is created. In recent years, because of the current small incisions, sagittal (parallel) slits can also give good angle control. Although angle control is good with both techniques, I still think that lateral slits provide slightly better and more consistent control. The early fears of vascular damage with lateral slits have not materialized, mainly as a consequence of the use of small blades, depth control, and tumescence before cutting. The other concern was that lateral slits would be more likely to transect preexisting hair. Minimizing transection of existing hair has more to do with the operator's ability to accurately judge the follicle's subcutaneous angle than choice of incisions. If the hair in the recipient area is shaved down to 2 mm, the exit angle of the recipient hair can be easily seen. Most of the time, because Asian hair is straight, the subcutaneous angle is the same as the exit angle; therefore, simply aligning the blade with the hair's exit angle is enough to minimize transections (Figs. 1, 2).

As Fig. 1 illustrates, the rapid directional changes at the center of the crown swirl becomes more gradual as we move further from the swirl. Lateral slits are slits cut perpendicular to the direction of hair flow. Because the slits are cut in rows they tend to form an arc or semicircular pattern. In an area of rapid directional changes, the arcs have small diameters. Lateral slits are also called coronal slits, but this is not an accurate description because "coronal" refers to an anatomical plane. Lateral slits have a variable direction and angle depending on where we are on the scalp. While cutting slits our focus needs to be on this hair direction and angle and nothing else, because the best cosmetic result comes when we get these parameters right.

Lateral slits (Fig. 3) are simple to do.

1. Point the handle of the blade holder in the same direction as the hair flow.
2. Lay the blade edge flat on the skin.

D. Pathomvanich and K. Imagawa (eds.), *Hair Restoration Surgery in Asians*
DOI 10.1007/978-4-431-99659-0_30, © Springer 2010

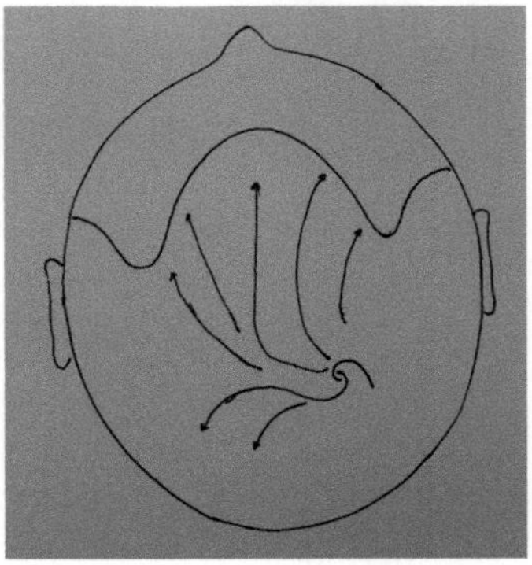

Fig. 1. The directional hair flow starting from the crown is shown

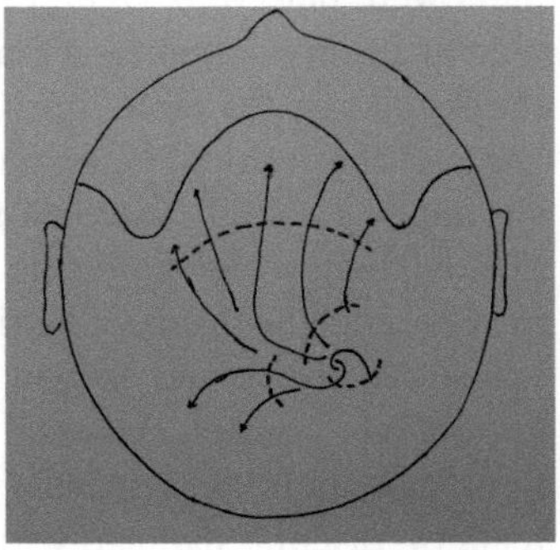

Fig. 2. *Dotted lines* represent lateral slits cut perpendicular to the direction of hair flow

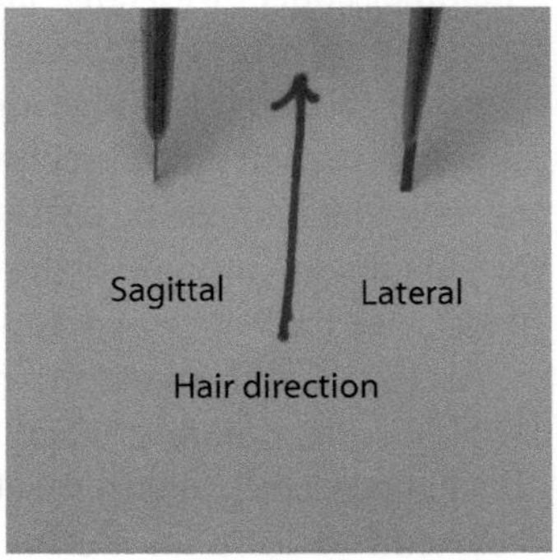

Fig. 3. Comparing lateral to sagittal cuts

3. Adjust the angle of the blade handle to match the subcutaneous follicular angle if there are existing hairs. Hair direction is usually obvious and can be seen if there are any miniaturized hair remaining. The challenge here is to align the blade with the existing follicle's subcutaneous angle to minimize transection. Most of the time the subcutaneous angle is the same as the exit angle, but sometimes the subcutaneous angle is often just slightly more vertical than the hair's exit angle and the blade may need to be slightly more vertical than the exit angle of the residual hair. Some surgeons will switch to parallel (sagittal)

incisions in areas of existing hair to try to minimize transections, but because Asian hair roots tend to splay below the surface, sagittal incisions may not have any advantage for minimizing transections. The key to minimizing transection is paying constant attention and adjusting the blade to match any changes in the direction and angle of the residual hair. This is not always easy to do.

When cutting slits, magnification is extremely important. There are multiple choices available, and the only way to choose is to try a few methods to see which one is the best fit. On follow-up visits, check to see if transection of residual hair has taken place. If the grafted hair has a halo of bare skin then the surrounding hair has been damaged. However, if fine residual hairs grow right up to the grafted hair, then little to no transection has taken place. Trying to minimize damage to residual hair is an ongoing challenge no matter what our skill level.

In areas of bare skin, where there are no residual hairs to dictate the blade angle, I generally use a 45° angle. In patients with limited donor hair, one trick to increase the apparent skin coverage is to lay the blade flatter to the skin surface to increase the hair's exit angle. Keeping the hair's exit angle closer to the skin increases the shingling effect and blocks more light from reaching the scalp. Lateral slits are excellent at producing acute angles and thus are especially suitable for areas such as the temples and eyebrows.

The same-sized blades used sagittally will make a longer slit on the skin than laterals; therefore, a slightly larger blade may be required when switching from sagittals to laterals. It will take time for both the surgeon and staff to adjust to this technique, and some surgeons use a combination of the two techniques. Many people do not see any cosmetic benefits to lateral slits, but it takes time to get really good with this technique and to realize its benefits. The person who does a few sessions of lateral slits and says "there is no difference" may be missing something that is really good. Despite a slow beginning, lateral slits are being adopted by more surgeons and are slowly becoming more mainstream. Casual feedback at meetings from those who have adopted this technique has been very encouraging.

A Debate over Premade Incisions Versus "Stick and Place"

J. Wong

Both premade incisions and "stick and place" are merely surgical techniques with advantages and drawbacks. The surgeon should use and become familiar with both techniques. Although the surgeon's skill and the surgical team's skill and experience play a more important role than any surgical technique per se, each technique does have unique advantages over the other in different circumstances. As we use premade sites most of the time, my perspective is biased toward premade sites. The stick-and-place method is currently used by some of the best surgeons producing excellent work.

1. Speed: in general, premade site are faster. Several years ago when comparing notes with Dr. David Seager (who practices mainly stick and plant), premade sites could save as much as 2 h for a 3000-graft case. Premade sites no longer have a speed advantage. Dr. Tykocinski and Dr. Rouston in Brazil use a two-person technique in which one person makes the slit with a custom blade, then turns the blade slightly sideways to open up the slit while a second person inserts the graft. Stick and place Brazil style is fast. We timed Dr. Tykocinsky's team inserting 800+ grafts per hour.
2. Spacing: premade sites are much more evenly spaced because they are made at the same time by one person. Because the sites are made by the same person the spacing is the same on both sides. In a two-person stick and place there are more chances for spacing variation because the two sides are made by different individuals.
3. Hair direction and angulation: premade sites have better and more consistent angle control.
4. Missed sites and piggy-backing (putting two grafts into one site): here the advantage goes to stick and place.
5. Working in long hair: with stick and place, there is no need to search for sites. The advantage goes to stick and place.
6. Ease of insertion: stick-and-place sites are a little easier to place because the blade both cuts and dilates the slit slightly.
7. Inserter's choice: in our clinic, the inserters vote in favor of premade sites because stick and place adds another step to their procedure and another instrument they need to hold. We have yet to try Dr. Tykocinski's two-person approach to stick and place, so this thinking may change.

D. Pathomvanich and K. Imagawa (eds.), *Hair Restoration Surgery in Asians*
DOI 10.1007/978-4-431-99659-0_31, © Springer 2010

Instead of debating which is better, the team should be proficient with both methods because each method brings its own strength and each clearly is better under different situations. I believe that in many other countries and in many states of the United States the assistants are not allowed to do stick and place, only the physician. This restriction might have an impact on those who relocate their practices.

Technique of Fast and Efficient Graft Insertion

J. Wong

Despite all the various mechanical implanting devices that have been tried in recent years, there is nothing yet that can rival the human hand using forceps. Our ability to do large densely packed sessions is dependent on having skilled technicians who can gently place grafts with speed. More cutters can always be added as needed, but only a maximum of two, or sometimes three, people can place at any one time. Consequently, the size of sessions is determined by the speed and skill of the placers. Too often, placing is done by the same three to four team members but ideally all the technicians should be trained to place grafts. The drawback to training new staff is that this slows down the surgery. If the training time is restricted to 30 min/day it will not slow the surgery down significantly, and if all the team members can place grafts it makes for a much more flexible team. Two quick placers will form the core of a very good team. Four quick placers will make an amazing team that can handle large cases and still finish in reasonable time. Inserter skill is the single most important factor determining surgical speed.

Time can also be saved if the surgery is planned to increase the team's overall efficiency. Once again, for 4000+ follicular unit (FU) sessions, leave the more time consuming areas such as the crown and temples, concentrating instead on the relatively large areas on the top extending from the hairline to the crown swirl. At the start of surgery, cut sufficient slits in the frontal third so that two people can plant at the front. If indicated, slits can also be cut further back just above the crown swirl, for a third planter. The idea is to space the sites out so that as many people as possible can insert at the same time. Because the slits are cut in rows, the planting can also be done in rows. Being methodical reduces the chances of missing slits or placing two grafts in the same slit. Placing is easier if we cut only what can be placed in 2 to 3 h because sites will often bleed a little more if left empty for too long.

Whenever possible, keep the graft supply close to the insertion site as this will minimize forceps travel time and allow the eyes to focus quicker. We also like to use finger bowls to keep the grafts moist and at the same time hold sufficient grafts to keep the planters busy for 5 to 10 min. This method minimizes the time spent turning around to obtain more grafts. The bowls that we use are homemade but there are many commercially available.

D. Pathomvanich and K. Imagawa (eds.), *Hair Restoration Surgery in Asians*
DOI 10.1007/978-4-431-99659-0_32, © Springer 2010

Fig. 1. Finger bowl

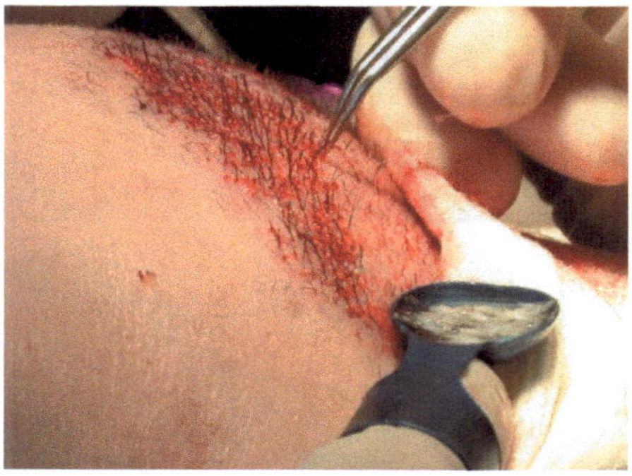

Fig. 2. Short and long nose insertion forceps

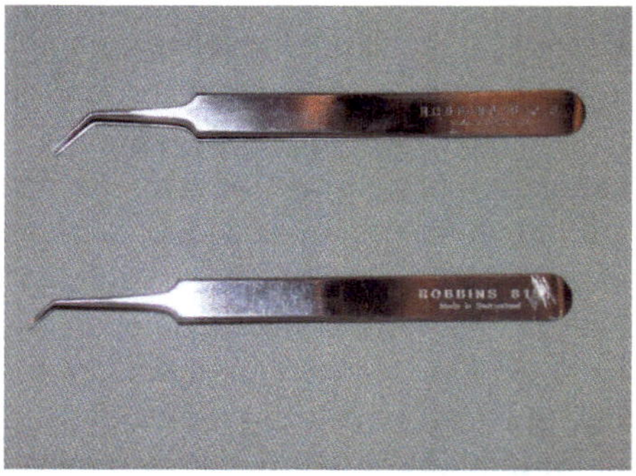

Prepared grafts are bunched in groups of 20 aligned in the same direction and placed on wet gauze in Petri dishes. This system makes it easier to keep track of the graft count and also allow the grafts to be placed in the finger bowls facing the same direction (Fig. 1). This arrangement saves some time as there is less need to spin grafts around before picking them up for insertion.

Lateral slits have a tighter fit and can be slightly more difficult to plant. One of our technicians likes to use a hook device (a 30 G needle bent at the tip) to open the slits before insertion. Our clinic uses the 815S forceps from Robbins Instruments. Robbins sells both the short- and long-tip type but we believe that the long-tip ones work the best (Fig. 2). These instruments are extremely delicate, and the tip can be easily damaged with handling and cleaning. Even slight tip damage will make insertion more difficult because the forceps will not release the graft cleanly. Small burrs on the tip can be smoothed away using a fine stone or a small needle holder. Oftentimes a malfunctioning forceps can turn an easy case into a difficult one, so always try a different forceps if difficulties are encountered. To minimize forceps damage we provide every technician with an individual forceps container, and most of the senior inserters have five to six planting forceps and two graft-cutting forceps to use at any one time. These forceps are not shared, and each person uses only their own instruments and is responsible for their cleaning and care. The damage rate has decreased significantly since we implemented this system.

For both surgeons and planters, there are few things more frustrating than after making 1000 to 1500 slits to have the techs tell you that the cuts are too shallow and the grafts are sticking out or that the slits are too small for the grafts. It is always a good idea at the start of surgery to do some test sites to ensure we have the correct blade size set at the proper depth. Slits deeper than what is required should also be avoided as this will produce more pitting. Popping grafts used to be a problem with the larger mini-grafts; with today's closely trimmed FU and custom-sized slits, popping is rarely seen.

Nearly all the patients coming to our clinic know about the shave and are prepared to live with it over the short term. Dense packing with premade sites up to around 3000 FU is quite manageable without shaving. If the plan is to do 4000+ FU then the recipient site needs to be shaved to work quickly and efficiently. Asians are very reluctant to shave but they are in fact good candidates because the recipient sites heal with minimal redness. Usually by 9 to 11 days after surgery, when the crusts in the recipient area are removed, there is very little to indicate that surgery has actually taken place. Most patients will be given a short haircut at 7 to 10 days post op to blend the short transplanted hair to the sides, and some people at this stage are comfortable enough to go without a hat.

Implanter

J.-C. Kim

Follicular unit transplantation uses the hair in their natural groupings. One of the great advantages of follicular unit transplantation is that a single session can stand completely on its own and look extraordinarily natural. Subsequent procedures are simply the decision of the patient to add additional density. However, this technique, with long operating time, reliance on a large surgical team, and use of more delicate grafts, introduces a new set of problems, all potentially manifesting as poor growth. The process of technique involves the joint efforts of highly trained and experienced assistants and the physician.

We have devised the KNU implanter. There are three types of KNU implanter: type L (equipped with an 18 G needle) for implanting three-hair follicular units, type M (20 G needle) for two-hair follicular units or single-hair grafts, and type S (22 G needle) for fine single-hair grafts (Fig. 1).

A follicular unit is placed onto the needle of the KNU implanter using jeweler's forceps (Fig. 2). The operator inserts the needle into the skin at the desired angle and pushes the plunger. The needle is automatically withdrawn, leaving the hair graft neatly tucked under the skin (Fig. 3). It should be noted that the small guide hook on the housing holds the hair graft in place while the needle is withdrawn. The guide hook on the implanter can make the epidermis level the same between grafts and recipient skin, so that the exit point of each hair looks very natural (Fig. 4). The KNU implanter may eliminate the crushing, squeezing, bending, piggybacking, and overmanipulation that can potentially reduce the graft survival rate. Making the proper direction and acute angle by using the KNU implanter is easier. An acute angle of insertion can reduce bleeding and the popping-up phenomenon. Follicular unit transplantation using the KNU implanter is especially suited to young patients or women who have general thinning because it allows the placing of grafts "in between" areas of thinning without removing a potentially long-lasting hair.

The patients require no bandage. The recipient area is always left open as this enables the transplanted area to be exposed to the air for drying.

We are routinely performing hair restoration sessions of approximately 3500 hair follicles (2000 grafts). Our operating time is about 3 to 4 h. We usually work

D. Pathomvanich and K. Imagawa (eds.), *Hair Restoration Surgery in Asians*
DOI 10.1007/978-4-431-99659-0_33, © Springer 2010

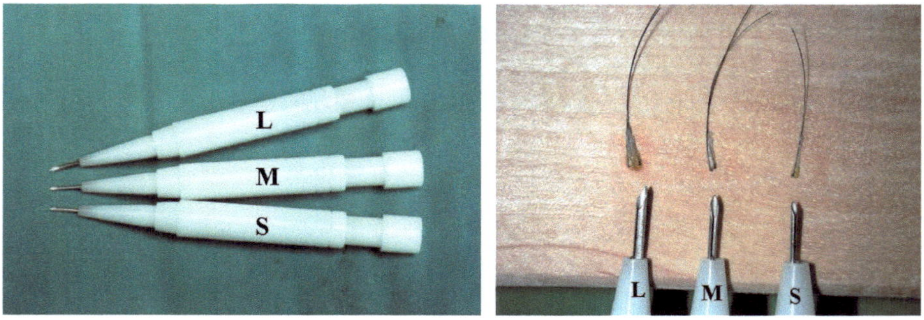

Fig. 1. Different sizes of KNU implanter (*left*) for different sizes of grafts (*right*). Types are described in text

Fig. 2. Loading a follicle into an implanter

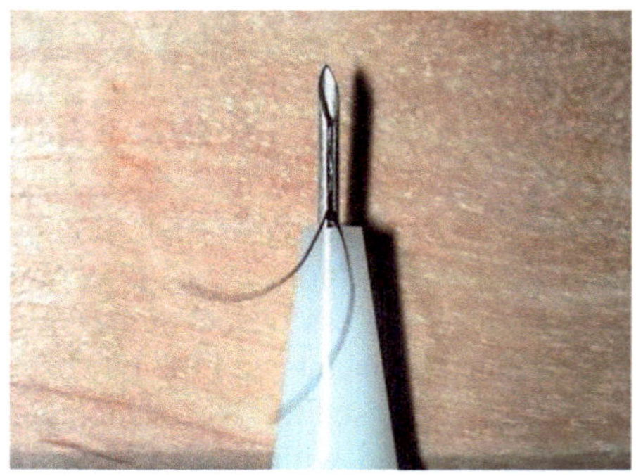

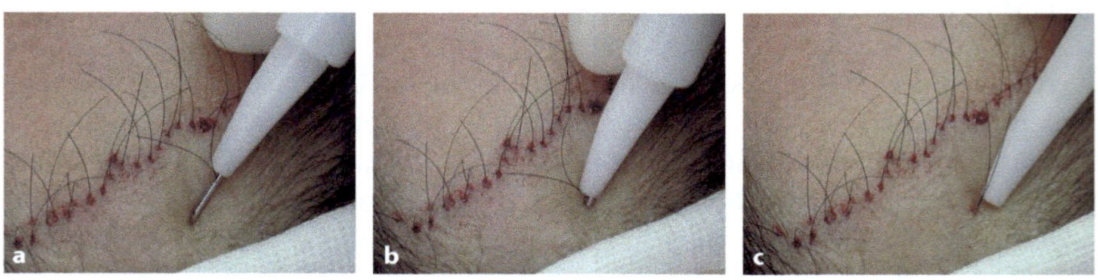

Fig. 3. Technique in using an implanter. **a** Needle is inserted in recipient skin. **b** The plunger is pushed. **c** The graft was tucked under the skin

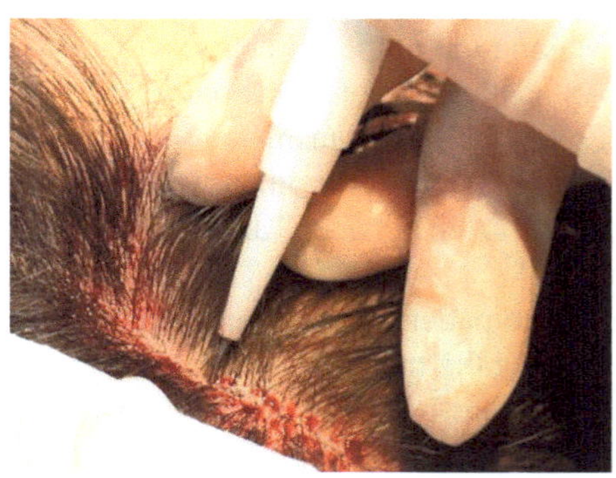

Fig. 4. Implanter can be used in the stick-and-place technique

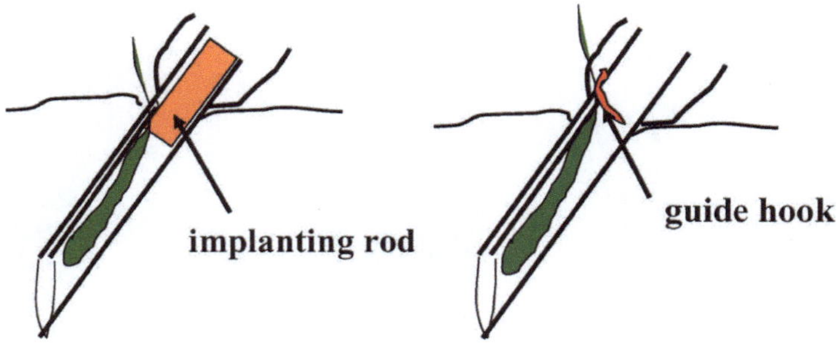

Fig. 5. A Choi implanter (*left*) and a KNU implanter (*right*)

as a six-person team: one doctor who implants follicular units, one assistant who inserts grafts into the needle of the KNU implanter, and four assistants who prepare the grafts.

Follicular unit grafting using the KNU implanter may be the most effective technique for Asians.

Part X
Hair Restoration in Women and Transsexual Males

Hair Restoration Surgery in Asian Women

M.J.K.S. Bunagan and D. Pathomvanich

Globally, hair loss negatively affects the lives of Asian women as it does women of other races [1,2]. In a study involving Caucasian women, those with highly visible hair loss reported a more negative impact on four dimensions (functioning, emotions, self-confidence, and stigmatization) compared with patients whose hair loss was only slightly visible [1]. This negative effect was similarly seen among Asian women in a study done in Singapore, which revealed that women with female pattern hair loss were socially embarrassed and "unhappy" about their condition [2]. For these aforementioned reasons, most patients in the Asian study sought treatment for their problem. Depending on the cause of hair loss, various treatment options are available. Although medical therapy is the treatment option for certain etiologies, for the other causes such as female pattern hair loss, hair transplantation may be a major consideration, especially with the newer techniques that lead to natural-looking results.

Asian women have particular hair characteristics that have to be taken into consideration when contemplating hair transplantation to attain the best cosmetic outcome. This chapter aims to provide information pertaining to hair transplantation in Asian women that may help the hair transplant surgeon to achieve the best results for this group.

Initial Consultation

Because hair loss in women is complex, it is essential that the cause of the hair loss be properly investigated to rule out etiologies that should be primarily treated medically and are not indications for hair transplantation. To establish the diagnosis, a thorough history and physical examination are essential. Laboratory testing should also be done as deemed necessary.

A common cause of hair loss in women is female pattern hair loss. One pattern among women is the Ludwig pattern where hair loss is confined primarily over the central and caudal portion of the scalp with retention of the frontal fringe of hair

D. Pathomvanich and K. Imagawa (eds.), *Hair Restoration Surgery in Asians*
DOI 10.1007/978-4-431-99659-0_34, © Springer 2010

over the hairline area [3]. Another pattern is the Norwood–Hamilton pattern in which the hair loss is mainly seen over the frontotemporal area, similar to the pattern seen in men [4,5]. Women may also have the Christmas tree or frontal accentuation pattern as described by Olsen, which starts as a widened hair part evolving into hair loss over the frontal and midline area [6]. Other causes of hair loss in women are telogen effluvium, postpartum hair loss, alopecia areata, trichotillomania, scarring alopecia caused by various dermatological diseases such as lichen planopilaris, frontal fibrosing alopecia, and lupus.

After the diagnosis is reached, treatment considerations may then be entertained. At this point, the decision as to whether hair transplantation would be a suitable option can be made. Hair transplantation should not be carried out in female patients whose hair loss is considered temporary following emotional stress, febrile illness, or childbirth. Other conditions that are not indications for hair transplantation are outlined below.

There are various indications for hair transplantation in women. Among Asian women, a retrospective study of 48 Asian female patients seen by Dr. Pathomvanich revealed that the main indications were female pattern hair loss (FPHL) at 59%, followed by scarring alopecia caused by burns, inactive disease, etc., at 16%, and cosmetic surgery-induced scars and alopecia at 14%. Among the patients with FPHL, the most common pattern was the Ludwig type at 36.3% followed by the Norwood–Hamilton pattern seen in 22.7% [7].

Hair Loss Etiologies *Not* Indicated for Hair Transplantation

- Telogen effluvium (resulting from endocrine causes, nutritional factors, psychological/physical stress, or drugs)
- Alopecia areata
- Active scarring alopecia (with perifollicular erythema or hyperkeratoses, considered a cicatricial alopecia variant)
- Trichotillomania

Hair Loss Etiologies that May Be Indications for Hair Transplantation

- Female pattern hair loss: Ludwig pattern, diffuse central thinning of the scalp with retention of the frontal fringe of the hairline
- Female pattern hair loss: Norwood–Hamilton pattern, mainly frontotemporal recession or without thinning over the vertex area
- Female pattern hair loss: Christmas tree pattern, frontal accentuation seen initially as a widened part, then may involve a broad area of the frontal hairline and the midline

- Cosmetic surgery-induced alopecia and scars (facelift, coronal lift, temporal lift, hair transplant with large grafts and flaps)
- Inactive scarring alopecia (scarring of the scalp from a burn such as hot oil, fire, acid)
- Pseudopelade and cicatricial alopecias inactive for several years

Preoperative Considerations in Asian Women

If the hair loss etiology is an indication for hair transplantation, the next step is to assess if the patient is a good candidate for this procedure. If there is diffuse thinning over the scalp, then the patient may not have sufficient donor hair to cover the hair loss at the recipient area. This situation should be discussed properly with the patient. This diffuse alopecia is more likely to occur in female patients than in males, as reflected in an Asian study [2].

For patients with FPHL, the application of minoxidil lotion is advised. This is the only medication currently approved by the U.S. Food and Drug Administration (FDA) for hair loss in women. The use of minoxidil is encouraged in conjunction with hair transplantation as this drug may help increase non-vellus hair counts and retard further thinning of existing hair.

For the effect of this drug among Asian women, the only clinical trial done was on the efficacy of 1% topical minoxidil versus placebo for androgenetic alopecia in Japanese female patients. The results showed a significant increase of non-vellus hair counts in the minoxidil group [8]. Several experimental studies have been undertaken on the efficacy of 2% minoxidil lotion among subjects with FPHL in the United States and in Europe, with the outcome revealing significant results over placebo [9,10]. Another study was conducted comparing 2% to 5% minoxidil lotion among female subjects with the 5% formulation showing statistical superiority over the 2% in the patient assessment of treatment benefit [11]. Various hair transplant surgeons such as Pathomvanich have used the 5% dosage among Asian female patients with good results.

A review should be done of all the medications that the patient is taking. Take particular note of drugs that may increase intraoperative bleeding, such as the anticoagulants, as well as aspirin and other nonsteroidal anti-inflammatory drugs (NSAIDS) [12]; even vitamin E has been implicated. Discontinuing aspirin for 7 days and NSAIDS for 3 days before the hair transplantation surgery is suggested [13]. Aside from conventional drugs, the intake of nonconventional medications such as herbal medicines should be questioned. Among Asian women there may be increased utilization of herbal supplements such as was seen in a study investigating complementary and alternative medicine use, including intake of herbal medications, which revealed that the highest level of use was among Asians [14]. Prescription of Chinese herbal medicines among Asians is also increasing [15]. Herbal drugs that may contain ginseng, ginger, gingko biloba, or other ingredients may potentially increase bleeding. Thus, it would be prudent to instruct the patient to stop these drugs about 1 week before the hair transplantation procedure.

The procedure and its possible complications, in general, would be similar to hair transplantation in men. However, in women it should be explained that there is a higher possibility of increased shedding of existing hair, which may occur several weeks to months after the transplantation procedure. Proper reassurance should be made that this condition is usually temporary and that the majority of the existing hair will grow back along with the transplanted hair. Women with a high count of vellus-type hair in the recipient region are especially at risk of permanent loss of density following transplantation.

For other general preoperative considerations common to both men and women, please refer to other chapters.

Hair Characteristics of Asian Women and Implications for the Hair Transplantation Procedure

In general, Asian women, as do Asian men, have medium-coarse, straight, black hair with a larger diameter, longer graft length, and lower follicular unit density than the hair of other racial groups.

In a study done on normal Chinese scalps, the female subjects had a mean of 71.7 follicular units (FU)/cm^2 over the occipital scalp and 86.6 FU/cm^2 over the frontal area, with an average of 70.78 FU/cm^2 overall [16]. In another study, Koreans had significantly lower densities compared to whites or blacks (although female subjects had a higher number of terminal hairs than the male subjects) [17]. In the Pathomvanich study of Asian female patients, the majority had densities ranging from 70 to 75 FU/cm^2, which, although lower than other races, still yielded adequate donor hair for the hair transplantation procedure [7]. In terms of hair restoration results, this lower follicular unit density count in Asian women is offset by the coarser hair that is characteristic of this group.

In these modern times, hairstyles of Asian women range from short to long, depending on the person's preference. Although the majority have straight hair, there are some who undergo artificial curling or perming. Some Asian women also undergo chemical hair dyeing to lighten the color of their hair. In the majority with straight hair, there may be less coverage than with wavy or curly hair because more light is reflected from the scalp. A lesser contrast between hair and skin color generally results in the appearance of thicker hair. Most Asians have black or dark brown hair, and this creates more contrast among those with light complexions, such as the Chinese, but would be less of a problem for darker-skinned Asians, such as the Indian or Malay populations. In addition, this contrast may be somewhat compensated by the larger hair diameter and relatively longer hair length in Asian women. These factors facilitate coverage of the underlying scalp. Because hair color, waviness, and length affect the cosmetic outcome of the hair transplantation procedure, all these various hair characteristics and styling options should be discussed with the patient to better enhance her postsurgical appearance.

With the aforementioned larger hair diameter and longer graft length seen in Asians, slit sizes in the recipient region are made with a relatively larger blade or hypodermic needle size as compared to those used for Caucasians. In the Pathomvanich study of Asian female patients, hypodermic needles of 20 or 21 G were mostly used for one-hair grafts and 18 or 19 G for two- or three-hair grafts during the hair transplantation procedure [7].

Approach to Hair Transplantation in Asian Women

In general, hair transplantation for Asian women (i.e., donor harvesting, graft preparation, slit creation, and insertion of grafts) follows the same procedure as that for men.

Donor harvesting of a woman's scalp is largely limited to the post-auricular and occipital area without extending to the temporal sides of the scalp. Hair over this area may become sparser and lead to visible scarring, especially when certain women's hairstyles are used.

In terms of grafts used in transplantation, follicular unit grafts with one, two, or three hairs are transplanted over the recipient area to achieve more natural-looking results [18]. Asian women have mostly follicular units with two hairs followed by one-hair FUs and three-hair FUs, as was seen in a Chinese study where the female subjects had 48.5% two-hair FUs, followed by 32.88% one-hair FUs and 16.36% three-hair FUs.[16] Depending on the type of hair loss manifested by the patient, these grafts can be used singly or paired to achieve the desired results; this is discussed further in the topics below.

In women, the hair loss usually involves a less extensive area, hence fewer grafts are needed for adequate hair restoration. In the Pathomvanich study, the female patients with a Ludwig pattern selected for restoration had an average 75 cm^2 hair loss, although this did not represent the entire thinning area. The mean graft number transplanted among these female patients was 1620 grafts at about 20–25 grafts/cm^2. Among the patients with Norwood–Hamilton pattern, the average hair loss area was 46 cm^2 and the average number of grafts transplanted was 1861 grafts at approximately 40 grafts/cm^2 [7].

In addition, depending on the type of hair loss problem, certain techniques are suggested for a particular indication, as discussed next.

Female Pattern Hair Loss

Ludwig Pattern (Fig. 1)

Because the main problem in this pattern is central thinning with retention of the frontal hairline, the goal is to add density over the thinning area.

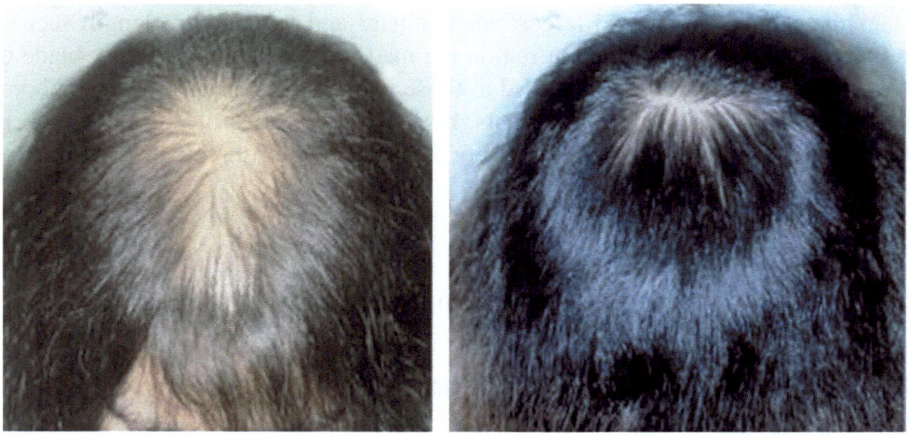

Fig. 1. Ludwig pattern of hair loss before (*left*) and after (*right*) transplantation of 1441 grafts

Points to consider are the following:

- The area to be transplanted has existing hair, so minimizing damage to these hair follicles is important. Adjacent hair follicle injury can be lessened by following the angle and direction of the existing hair [18] as well as by using hypodermic needles rather than the sharper mini-blades when creating slits.
- Adding additional density to areas with thinning hair can be achieved with transplant densities of 20–25 FU/cm^2 as there are still hairs present and Asian women have larger-diameter hairs, which adds to the illusion of increased density.
- Asian women usually have a significant number of one-hair FUs, so pairing of these individual FUs when transplanting will maximize the appearance of density.
- In women who have a hair parting preference, more FUs can be transplanted along the part side and fewer over the non-part side to create the illusion of greater density.
- With the existing hairs present in this pattern, premade slits may be hard to find; thus, utilizing more of the "stick-and-place" technique may speed up the transplantation process.

Norwood-Hamilton Pattern (Fig. 2)

The most common Norwood–Hamilton pattern seen among the Asian women in the Pathomvanich study was loss in the frontotemporal recession; thus, the goal would be to restore the frontal hairline by filling in the frontotemporal corners [7].

Points to consider are the following:

- Planning the shape of the feminine hairline with the patient's input is crucial (oval, heart shape, with or without widow's peak, etc.). This plan includes atten-

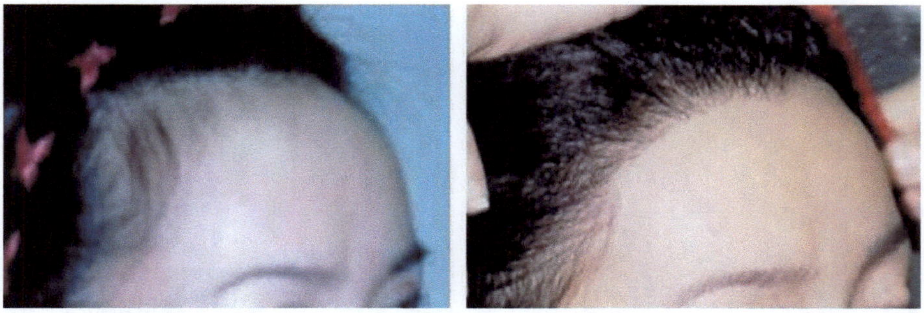

Fig. 2. Norwood–Hamilton pattern of hair loss, before (*left*) and after (*right*) transplantation of 989 grafts

tion to whether the temples will be involved, because hair over the temple area more commonly points in an inferior or posterior direction and is angled acutely.

- Because this is a highly visible area, making the transplanted hair as natural looking as possible is important. This can be achieved by transplanting all follicular unit grafts (FUGs) starting with one-hair FUGs at the very front (transition zone from forehead to hairline) and then two- to three-hair FUGs further back.
- For this pattern, there is usually almost total loss of terminal hair over the frontotemporal area. Even if hairs still exist, they are usually vellus hair. Thus to adequately restore the highly visible frontotemporal hairline the density goal is higher compared to the Ludwig pattern, ranging from 30 to 40 FU/cm^2 or even 50 FU/cm^2 in suitable candidates.
- Minimal to nonexistent terminal hairs are present; thus, aside from hypodermic needles, sharper mini-blades may be utilized to create premade slits.

Scars and Alopecia Resulting from Cosmetic Surgery (Fig. 3)

The most common cosmetic procedures that may result in inadvertent scarring and alopecia are conventional facelifts, coronal lifts, and temporal lifts. Please refer to other chapters for details.

Scarring Alopecia Caused by Burns or Inactive Disease

For patients with scarring alopecia resulting from disease, the condition must have been inactive for at least a few years before hair transplantation can even be considered. Active or recurring disease may cause destruction of the new transplants. It is not always easy to prove inactivity, and one should never accept that patient's

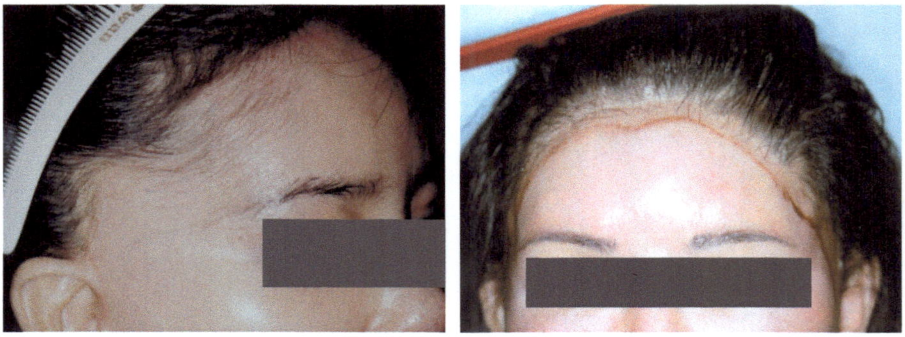

Fig. 3. Candidates for hair transplant: scarring alopecia from facelift

word on the subject. Serial photographs taken over a 2-year period and biopsies from the regions of last known activity are essential. If the disease is truly inactive, then hair transplantation can be undertaken with satisfactory results, although the patient should be warned of the possibility of later recurrence.

Points to consider are the following:

- In areas with scarring, there is a limited vascular supply, so it is wise to transplant at a lesser density, such as 20 FU/cm^2, over the alopecic area.
- It must be explained to the patient that, although the transplanted density will be much lower than the surrounding hair, this outcome will still be fairly adequate to cover the area that has scarring.
- For natural-looking results, the angle and direction of the hairs adjacent to the alopecic area should be followed.

References

1. Schmidt S, Fischer TW, Chren MM, et al (2001) Strategies of coping and quality of life in women with alopecia. Br J Dermatol 144:1038–1043
2. Goh CL (2002) A retrospective study on the characteristics of androgenetic alopecia among Asian races in the National Skin Centre, a tertiary dermatological referral centre in Singapore. Ann Acad Med Singap 31:751–755
3. Ludwig E (1977) Classification of the types of androgenetic alopecia (common baldness) occurring in the female sex. Br J Dermatol 97:247–254
4. Hamilton JB (1951) Patterned loss of hair in man: types and incidence. Ann N Y Acad Sci 53:708–728
5. Norwood OT (1975) Male pattern baldness: classification and incidence. South Med J 68:1359–1365
6. Olsen EA (2001) Female pattern hair loss: clinical features and potential hormonal factors. J Am Acad Dermatol 45:s70–s80.
7. Pathomvanich D, Bunagan K (2008) Hair transplantation in Asian women: a retrospective review of common indications, procedural techniques and post-operative outcomes. Poster presentation at the International Society of Hair Restoration Surgery annual meeting

8. Tsuboi R, Tanaka T, Nishikawa T, et al (2007) A randomized, placebo-controlled trial of 1% topical minoxidil solution in the treatment of androgenetic alopecia in Japanese women. Eur J Dermatol 17:37–44
9. Jacobs JP, Szpunar CA, Warner ML (1993) Use of topical minoxidil therapy for androgenetic alopecia in women. Int J Dermatol 32:758–762
10. DeVillez RL, Jacobs JP, Szpunar CA, et al (1994) Androgenetic alopecia in the female. Treatment with 2% topical minoxidil solution. Arch Dermatol 130:303–307
11. Lucky AW, Piacquadio DJ, Ditre CM, et al (2004) A randomized, placebo-controlled trial of 5% and 2% topical minoxidil solutions in the treatment of female pattern hair loss. J Am Acad Dermatol 50:541–553
12. Goldsmith S, Leshin B, Owen J (1993) Management of patients taking anticoagulants and platelet inhibitors prior to dermatologic surgery. J Dermatol Surg Oncol 19:578–581
13. Unger W (2004) Pre-operative preparation and instructions. In: Unger W, Shapiro R (eds) Hair transplantation, 4th edn. Dekker, New York, pp 189–190
14. Arcury TA, Suerken CK, Grzywacz JG, et al (2006) Complementary and alternative medicine use among older adults: ethnic variation. Ethnic Dis 16:723–731
15. Hsieh SC, Lai JN, Lee CF, et al (2008) The prescribing of Chinese herbal products in Taiwan: a cross-sectional analysis of the national health insurance reimbursement database. Pharmacoepidemiol Drug Saf 17:609–619
16. Tsai RY, Lee SH, Chan HL (2002) The distribution of follicular units in the Chinese scalp: implications for reconstruction of natural-appearing hairlines in Orientals. Dermatol Surg 28:500–503
17. Lee HJ, Ha SJ, Lee JH, et al (2002) Hair counts from scalp biopsy specimens in Asians. J Am Acad Dermatol 46:218–221
18. Unger WP, Unger RH (2003) Hair transplanting: an important but often forgotten treatment for female pattern hair loss. J Am Acad Dermatol 49:853–860

Hair Restoration Surgery in Transsexual Males

D. Pathomvanich

Good results and low cost have made Thailand the most attractive country in the world in providing sexual reassignment surgery (SRS).

Incidence

The incidence of SRS in Caucasians is low and has been estimated at between 1:5000 and 1:50000 [1]. The incidence may be very high, around 1:15000, in Asians, according to a few prominent plastic surgeons who have performed SRS in Thailand. There is no report in the literature about the incidence of SRS specifically in Asians.

Female to Male Transgender/Transsexual Female

In our practice, we have not encountered anyone of this group.

Male to Female Transgender/Transsexual Male

The incidence and terminology of this group were well reported by Richard Shiell [2]. Obviously, appropriate psychiatrist evaluation is important before surgery, but most of those requesting sex change would have considered themselves women since childhood.

Asians who underwent SRS were generally younger (18–35 years) than the Caucasian counterparts (30–70 years), according to Dr. Preecha Tiewtranon, who has performed the largest number of SRS in Thailand.

D. Pathomvanich and K. Imagawa (eds.), *Hair Restoration Surgery in Asians*
DOI 10.1007/978-4-431-99659-0_35, © Springer 2010

Those who already have SRS, or are in the process of having SRS, are usually on female hormone pills with or without finasteride, dutasteride, or minoxidil lotion. The majority of Asians who present to our clinic are Norwood male pattern baldness (MPB) class III, in comparison to class III–VI in the Caucasian counterparts. They may have received, or are planning to receive, multiple cosmetic procedures such as nasal augmentation, chin implant, zygomatic bone reduction, liposuction, removal of prominent frontal bone, and breast augmentation. Restoring a feminine hairline is obviously part of the list.

It is not uncommon for the patients to squeeze in various operations during their short stay in Thailand. They want to complete every procedure to look good and return to work with minimal cosmetic disfigurement. The hair surgeons must take into consideration the time restraint. Caution must be taken in scheduling lengthy mega-sessions as the patients may already have extensive blood loss from multiple procedures. The limited stay of the tourist-patient, however, will not allow the procedures to be scheduled too far apart. Most patients are reluctant to pay the travel expense to return on a later date for further surgery.

Although hair transplantation can be safely performed soon after SRS or other cosmetic surgery, one must bear in mind that on occasions the patients may not be able to proceed. The pain after breast augmentation, abdominal liposuction, or tummy tuck may render them unable to lie prone for donor harvesting. However, to my surprise, most patients tolerated the procedure very well despite pain and discomfort from other cosmetic surgery and SRS.

Surgeons should be aware that there may be a higher incidence of human immunodeficiency virus (HIV) positivity in this group of patients, and extra precautions should be taken even if a blood test is negative.

Designing the Hairline

One good thing in operating on male transsexuals who undergo SRS is that the hair loss has usually ceased consequent to estrogen treatment, finasteride, or past orchidectomy. Sometime even a little hair growth can be gained from the female hormone pill. All the patients want to have a feminine hairline. They hate the square shape or temple recession typically seen in men. Many already have the design in mind, and some bring along women's magazines to show the hairline they want.

I place the first dot at each temple point, a second one at mid-frontal, and the third one at mid-temple. In connecting the dots, an oval-shaped hairline is drawn to close the temple, with or without a widow's peak, according to their preferences. With the aid of the new laser beam device, a symmetrical hairline can be designed and created in just a minute [3]. Irregularities are then added onto the hairline to create a natural appearance. Because most Asian patients undergo their sex change at an early age, they present with minimal baldness, mostly Norwood II–III (see Fig. 1); this means that the surgery can be completed in just one pass and the overall result is good. Those who demand very high density may return at a later date for more sessions.

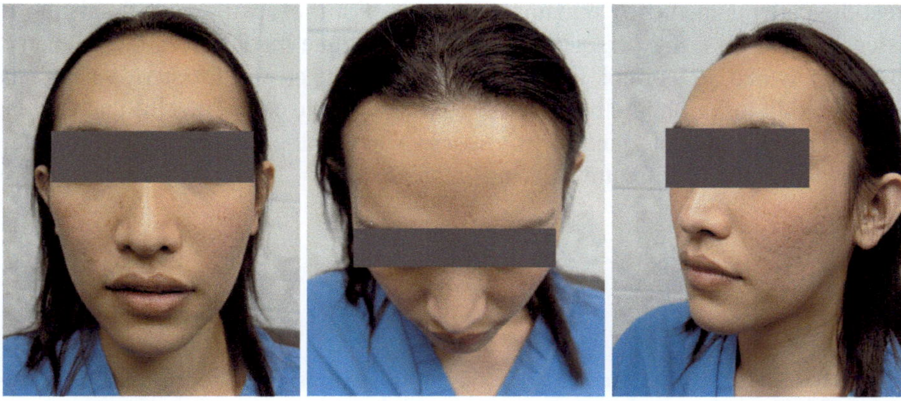

Fig. 1. Preoperative photograph, 29-year-old transsexual male

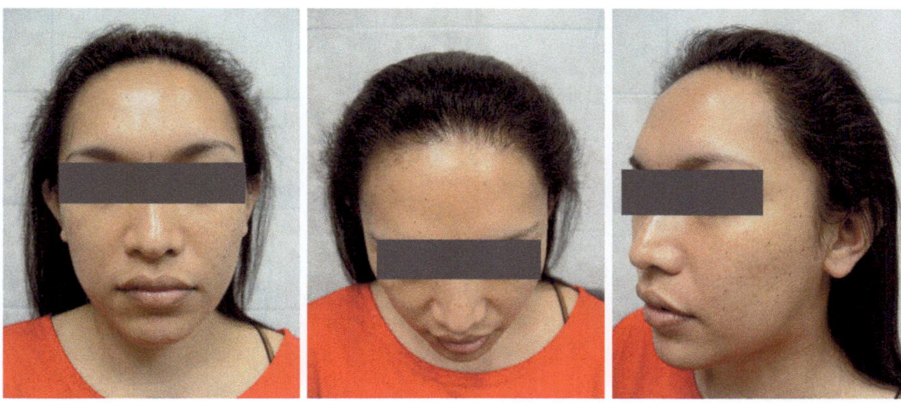

Fig. 2. Postoperative photograph taken after 8 months, 2138 follicular unit grafts were transplanted

Technique

The technique of the transplant is basically the same as described in the chapter on the recipient site. Donor hair is selected from mid-occiput at the supranuchal ridge. With trichophytic donor closure, the scar is almost invisible.

Medical Treatment

Theoretically, once the greatest source of testosterone is removed by SRS, hair loss should stop despite the small amount secreted by the adrenal gland. Whether to treat the patients medically remains a dilemma. For those with a family history of extensive hair loss, my personal feeling is to continue medical treatment whether they already had SRS or not. If there is thinning in the crown, finasteride 1 mg plus 5% minoxidil lotion should be taken for at least a year to counteract the testosterone secreted by the adrenal gland. Yearly assessment can then be carried out to determine whether medical treatment is still indicated.

References

1. Walinder J (1971) Incidence and sex ratio of transsexualism in Sweden. Br J Psychiatry 119:195–196
2. Shiell RC (2004) Hair transplant in the transsexual male. In: Hair transplantation, 4th edn. Dekker, New York, pp 602–606
3. Pathomvanich D, Bertram Ng (2008) Laser assisted hairline placement. Hair Transplant Forum International 18(5)

Part XI
Repairs: Personal Techniques

Repair of Iatrogenic Scarring and Non-Scarring Alopecia from Cosmetic Surgery

D. Pathomvanich

Alopecia from Temporal Lift, Facelift, and Coronal Lift

Patients with aged-looking faces continue to seek cosmetic surgery to correct unwanted wrinkles, loose neck skin, and brow ptosis. It is beyond doubt that cosmetic surgery improves the sagging skin, but at the risk of an unsightly scar, potential hair loss, or a misplaced sideburn.

After a mid-facelift the sideburns are usually misplaced and pulled to a more upward position. Absence of the sideburns from where they should be will expose the scar from the lift. Such a scar is more noticeable when the surgeons make the incision anterior to the temple hair line (pretrichial). Even if the incision is made within the temple hair (post-trichial), it may still become wide and visible through the temple hair. For temporal lift, the pull from the Russian thread also elevates the temple hairline and misplaces the sideburns to a higher position.

A conventional forehead lift often results in a wide scar across the scalp from ear to ear. Some patients are disturbed with this appearance as they can no longer wear the hair short without exposing the scar. In the worst scenario, the good hair does not return anterior to the incision. The final result can be both scarring and non-scarring alopecia, together with a deformed hairline and a high forehead. Sometimes the hair loss also occurs at the temples. All these events are detrimental to the patient's self-confidence. Fortunately, a properly performed endoscopic forehead lift, in good hands, can result in minimal if any scarring, and with minimal or no hair loss [1,2].

Repair to Scars Resulting from Facelifts and Temporal Lifts

Timing of the repair is crucial. The patient should wait a minimum of 6 months after surgery to give a chance for the lost hair to grow back and for the scar to mature. One can presume the hair loss is permanent if there is no growth after 6 months. Hair restoration surgery is then indicated to replace the loss and camouflage the scar.

D. Pathomvanich and K. Imagawa (eds.), *Hair Restoration Surgery in Asians*
DOI 10.1007/978-4-431-99659-0_36, © Springer 2010

Repairing Scars Following the Temporal Lift

Pretrichial Scars

The hair must be grafted anterior to and within the white scar. If only the scar is transplanted, its shininess is still obvious with minimal cosmetic improvement. The new hairline should be irregular with the single-hair grafts directed inferiorly and posteriorly to camouflage the scar. Usually the scar is straight with a short distance from the temporal to the brow and lateral canthus. Transplanting too far anteriorly from the scar will make the temple too close to the eye and create a poor cosmetic look.

Post-trichial Scars

One can simply insert grafts within the scar.

For Those with Russian Thread Lift

The new hairline should extend to restore the lower temple hairline and sideburn if indicated. The procedure is rather straightforward as described in Chapter 43 on transplanting sideburn.

Repairing Conventional Forehead Lift

Post-trichial Incision

The incision behind the hairline can lead to a wide scar as well as hair loss if excessive skin is excised. The temple scar also tends to be wider.

The scar can be revised by excision followed by trichophytic closure [3–5] or W-plasty [6]. If there is no cosmetic improvement, one can fill the scar with hair grafts. There is no firm consensus regarding direction of the transplanted hair. Some surgeons plant parallel to the scar, others are directed across the scar. All methods seem to give good cosmetic results.

The original hairline moves upward after the lift and creates a high forehead. In some, this may be associated with thinning hair anterior to the scar. To regain a more youthful appearance a lower hairline needs to be constructed. It is important to design a feminine hairline for women. Some patients prefer to have a widow's peak while others may want the anteriormost point to be round, a U-shape, or an inverted U-shape.

As it is very difficult to achieve symmetry on the two sides, the distance from the temple point to the eyebrow must be measured to ensure that both temporal points lie in the same coronal plane. With the introduction of the cross-beam laser, a symmetrical hairline can now be easily drawn (see laser-assisted hairline placement). Irregularities are then added to achieve a natural look.

The area is then measured in square centimeters (cm^2) and converted to a number of grafts by the Chang method [7]. At least 40–50 grafts/cm^2 are needed at the front top, and less at the temporal and sideburn regions.

The procedure will take longer than the usual scalp hair transplantation. First, it involves many areas including the sideburn, temple, and forehead on both sides. The surgeon must plan which area should be transplanted first to shorten the procedure. Also, it is difficult to have three assistants inserting the grafts simultaneously because of the position of the patient. I usually premake incisions at the frontal and part of the frontotemporal regions before asking the patient to lie on the side. One assistant will then insert grafts into the premade incisions, while another assistant sticks and places grafts in the temple and sideburn at the same time. On completion, the patient turns the face to the other side and the process is repeated in the same fashion. The surgeon might choose to premake all incisions before insertion, but this is more time consuming, in my experience.

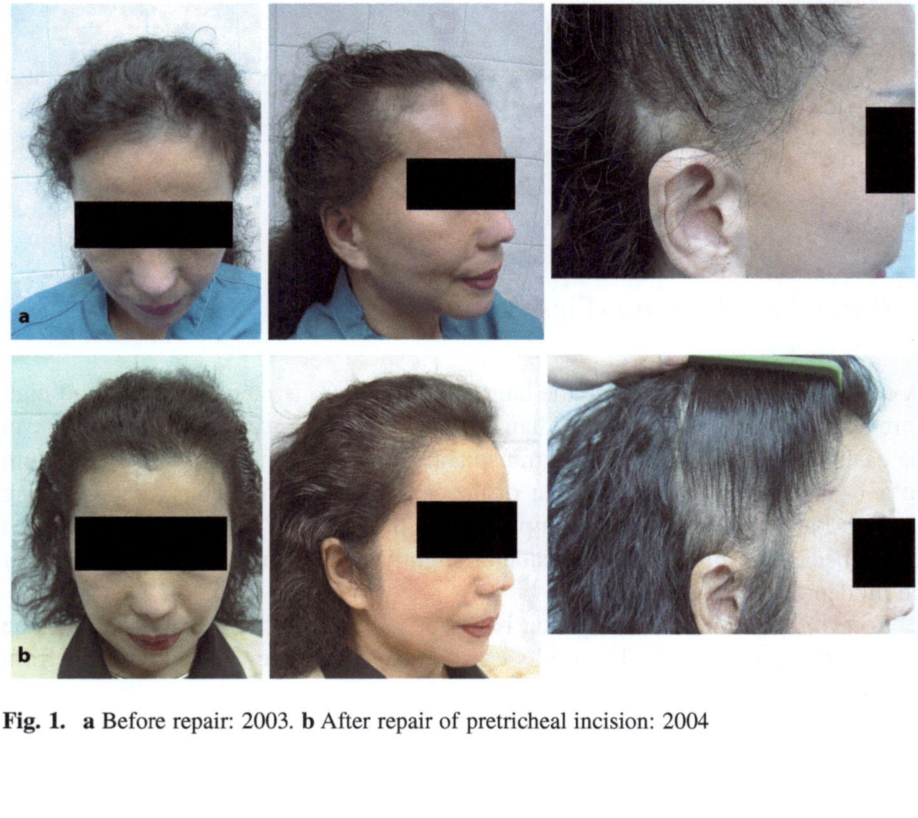

Fig. 1. **a** Before repair: 2003. **b** After repair of pretricheal incision: 2004

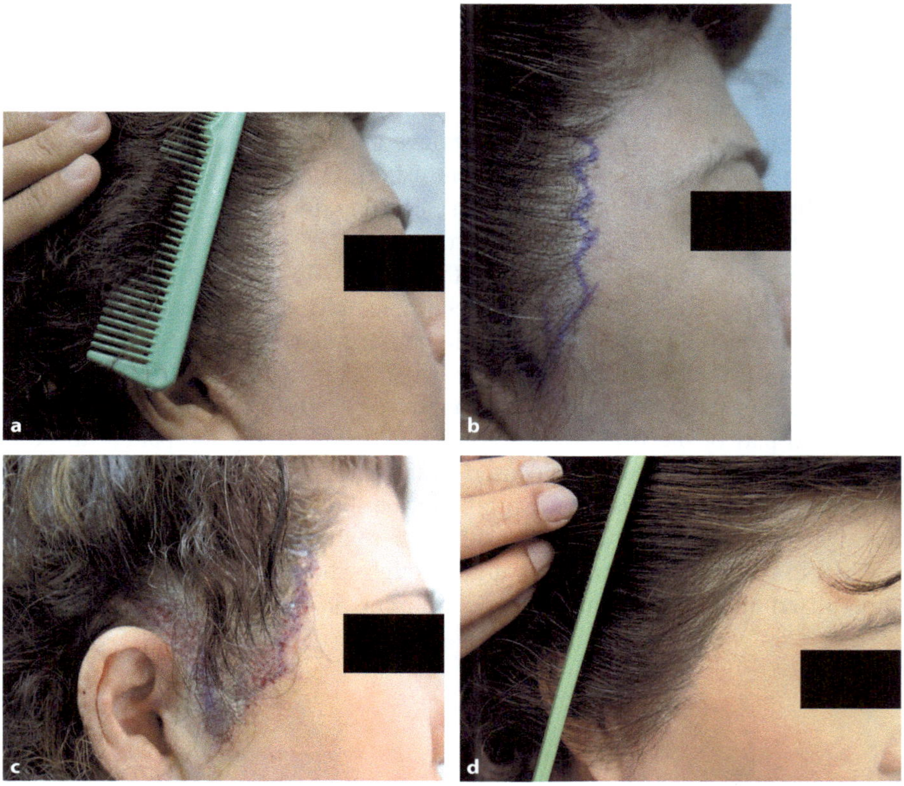

Fig. 2. **a** Scar from temporal lift. **b** The area is outlined with gentian violet. **c** Immediately after transplant. **d** Postoperative result

A Pretricheal Incision (Figs. 1, 2)

A coronal lift does not elevate the hairline. Also, there is no hair loss and no high forehead. However, the narrowed hairline may reveal the scar. Any scar if high can be easily be camouflaged by hair transplantation. Grafts should cover a minimum of a 1-cm zone anterior to the scar or the scar will remain visible when combing the hair backward; this becomes a problem if the forehead is very narrow. In such cases, because the transplant is inside or slightly beyond the scar, the latter cannot be hidden completely.

To avoid a pretrichial white scar, hair grafts should be transplanted at the same time as the temporal lift. The grafts can be taken from the excised scalp or from the occiput.

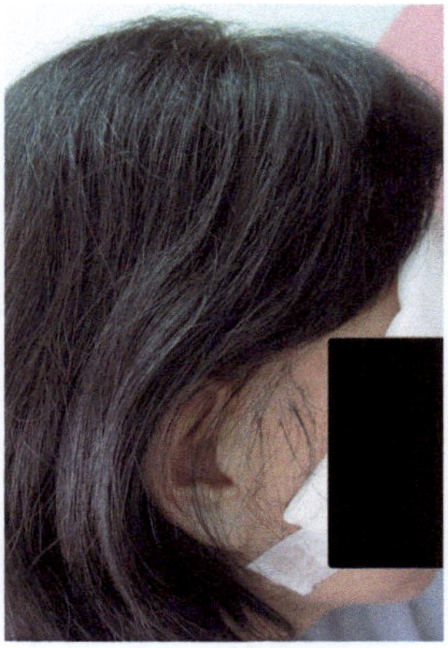

Fig. 3. Patient who has side-burn transplant with mini-grafts

Repairing Facelift with Temporal Lift

The sideburn is misplaced and needs reconstruction. The scar at the temple is usually wide and also requires transplantation (see Fig. 3).

References

1. Niamtu J III (2006) Endoscopic brow and forehead lift: a case for new technology. J Oral Maxillofac Surg 64:1129–1132
2. De Cordier BC, de la Torre JI, Al-Hakeem MS, et al (2002) Endoscopic forehead lift: review of technique, cases, and complications. Plast Reconstr Surg 110:1558–1568
3. Frechet P (2005) Donor harvesting with invisible scar. Hair transplant Forum Int 15:119–120

Cicatricial Alopecia in Hair Transplantation

D. Pathomvanich

The hair of the scalp is a human characteristic that conveys aspects of self-image, identity, and health. Hair loss from disease or other conditions may result in disturbed self-perception and psychological conflicts. Cicatricial alopecia encompasses a diverse group of disorders characterized by permanent destruction of the hair follicles and irreversible hair loss. It is classified into primary and secondary cicatricial alopecia [1].

In primary cicatricial alopecia, the hair follicle is the main target. There is destruction of follicular epithelium and or its associate adventitial dermis with relative sparing of the interfollicular reticular dermis [2–4], e.g., lichen planopilaris (LPP), folliculitis decalvans, discoid lupus erythematosus, frontal fibrosing alopecia, dissecting folliculitis/cellulitis, and pseudopelade of Brocq.

Secondary cicatricial alopecia is a nonfollicular disease that indirectly causes follicular destruction, e.g., from trauma, burn, chemical processing from dyes, curling or straightening, infection, syphilis, tuberculosis (TB), radiodermatitis, or benign or malignant tumor. In primary cicatricial alopecia, the cause and pathogenesis of many of the disorders are largely unknown.

Dermatological disorders causing permanent hair loss such as cicatricial alopecia make immediate diagnosis and therapeutic intervention imperative. Diagnostic hallmarks for all forms of cicatricial alopecia are as follows:

- Visible loss of the follicular ostia
- Destruction of the hair follicle on histopathological examination [5]

Location of the biopsy is very important: it should include part of the hair and the lesion. At least two specimens, 4 mm each, should be sent for horizontal and vertical section and direct immunofluorescence.

For primary cicatricial alopecia, the appropriate time for corrective surgery is still debated; a minimum of 2 years after diagnosis is acceptable to the majority of surgeons. Biopsy of the lesion before grafting is essential. The patient must be informed that if the disease recurs, the hair will be lost. The majority of patients who have cicatricial alopecia will be seen and treated first by a dermatologist. Hair transplant surgeons will get a referral from their colleagues when hair loss is not improved over a period of time and the patient wants to have his or her hair restored.

D. Pathomvanich and K. Imagawa (eds.), *Hair Restoration Surgery in Asians*
DOI 10.1007/978-4-431-99659-0_37, © Springer 2010

Secondary cicatricial alopecia, the type increasingly seen in hair transplant offices, most often results from facial cosmetic surgery, such as temporal and coronal lift or direct brow lift (see Chapter 35), and less often from a burn injury, which was commonly seen in the past.

The surgical technique is the same as hair transplantation for male pattern baldness, but often no dense packing or multiple sessions are required [6].

The timing of repair is crucial for secondary cicatricial alopecia. A minimal waiting period of 4 to 6 months is recommended, to be assured that there will be no further hair growth and that the scar is mature.

The strategies for repair are the following:

1. Excise the scar if the lesion is small. Use serial excisions if the lesion is moderate in size.
2. Hair transplantation alone [7,8] or in combination with scar reduction.
3. Tissue expansion and reconstruction of the defect [9].
4. Scalp flap [10].

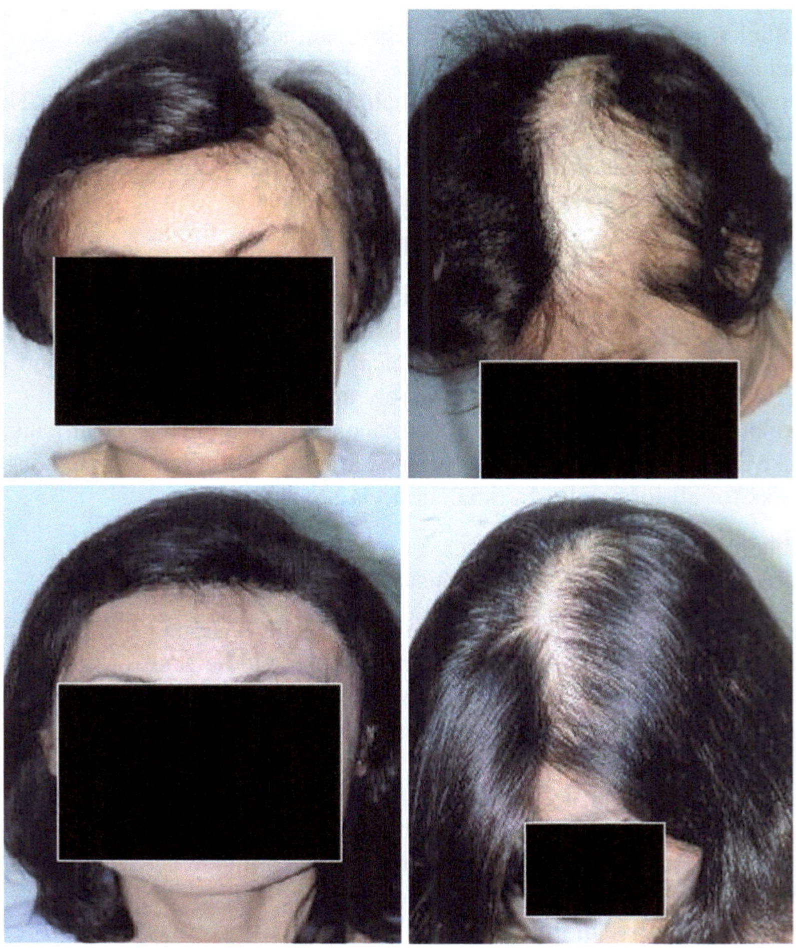

The scar should be evaluated with regard to the size, thickness, and skin texture. Alternative options must be discussed with the patient. Some hair surgeons may do only hair grafting while others solely use tissue expansion together with scar excision. Both tissue expansion and scar repair demand skill and experience from the surgeon. The surgeon must decide the technique that is best and that will benefit the patient.

If the area involved is extensive, a hairpiece may be the only option. The hairpiece, however, can be camouflaged by reconstructing the hairline with hair grafts. Although the technique is the same, the scar is usually thin and may not be able to accommodate the grafts. Brandy recommended cutting back with a Nokor needle or creating pockets in which to place the grafts. Injecting tumescence fluid immediately before making the slit can be helpful. The grafts should not be densely packed because of the poor blood supply. Multiple sessions are usually needed.

Figure 1 shows scarring alopecia from hot oil spillage since childhood: Fig. 1a is preoperative, Fig. 1b is 7 months postoperative, first session, and Fig. 1c is postoperative, 1 year after the second session.

The picture shows pseudopelade of Brocq. The patient had one session of hair transplantation but did not return for a follow-up. She wrote a letter stating the hairs were growing well but needed to increase in density.

References

1. Somani N, Bergfeld WF (2008) Cicatricial alopecia: classification and histopathology. Dermatol Ther 21(4):221–237
2. Otberq N, Wu WY, McElwee KJ, Shapiro J (2008) Diagnosis and management of primary cicatricial alopecia: part I. Skin Med 7(1):19–26
3. Headington JT (1996) Cicatricial alopecia. In: Whiting DA (ed) Update on hair disorders. Saunders, Philadelphia, pp 773–782
4. Alzolibani AA, Kang H, Otberg N, et al (2008) Pseudopelade of Broq. Dermatol Ther 21(4):257–263
5. Sperling LC, Cowper SE (2006) The histopathology of primary cicatricial alopecia. Semin Cutan Med Surg 25(1):41–50
6. Unger W, Unger R, Wesley C (2008) The surgical treatment of cicatricial alopecia. Dermatol Ther 21(4):295–311
7. Brandy DA (1993) The exclusive use of slit mini-micrografting for the correction of a large frontoparietal scalp defect. Am J Cosmet Surg 10:112–115
8. Kwon OS, Kim MH, Park SH, et al (2007) Staged hair transplantation in cicatricial alopecia after carbon dioxide laser-assisted scar tissue remodeling. Arch Dermatol 143:457–460
9. Wang SC, Chen FL, Li JY (1991) Soft tissue expansion in the treatment of scar alopecia in preschool children. Chin Med J 104:164–167
10. Takatoshi Y, Watanabe Y, Yamashita K, et al (2002) New treatment of a visible linear scar in the scalp: multiple hair-bearing flap technique. Br J Plast Surg 55(4):324–329

The Repair of Unwanted Plugs

D. Pathomvanich

There continue to be unhappy patients entering a hair transplant clinic with large punch grafts that were transplanted before 1990. With progressive hair loss, these plugs stand out and become unsightly. Although some of the plugs can be salvaged, those patients with extensive hair loss, a very low hairline, and minimal donor hair always challenge the skill of the hair transplant surgeon.

The patients must be informed what can and cannot be done to have a realistic expectation.

Strategy for the Repair

There are many methods of repair to improve the cosmetic outcome of the plug [1–4]. The surgeon has to carefully select the option to meet the individual's needs.

1. Partial or complete excision of the individual plug and then recycling the grafts (see Fig. 2).
2. Row excision of the plugs.
3. Add on density among the plugs.
4. Reconstruct a hairline using single-hair grafts to camouflage the plugs (see Fig. 3).
5. Reduce the size of the bald area by excision.
6. Remove the unwanted hair and resurface the scar with laser.

Some patients may prefer just to shave off all the plugs. Unfortunately, the scars from the plugs are still obvious to the naked eye.

Plugs in the Front

My approach is to excise the first two rows in the front and then recycle the grafts. Any unsightly individual plugs are also removed. Large plugs of 4–5 mm are dissected into follicular unit grafts.

D. Pathomvanich and K. Imagawa (eds.), *Hair Restoration Surgery in Asians*
DOI 10.1007/978-4-431-99659-0_38, © Springer 2010

For small plug grafts 2–3 mm in size placed high in the frontal area, a new hairline can be reconstructed at least 1.5 to 2 cm below the plugs to hide the corn row. The patient in Fig. 1 had small plugs but did not want them removed. A new hairline was constructed with add-on density. Despite a good cosmetic improvement, the small plugs are still visible. These undesired plugs can be partially debulked to create a more natural look.

For those with a very low hairline, progressing to class VI–VII, and with minimal donor availability, the best option is to remove the existing hairline grafts

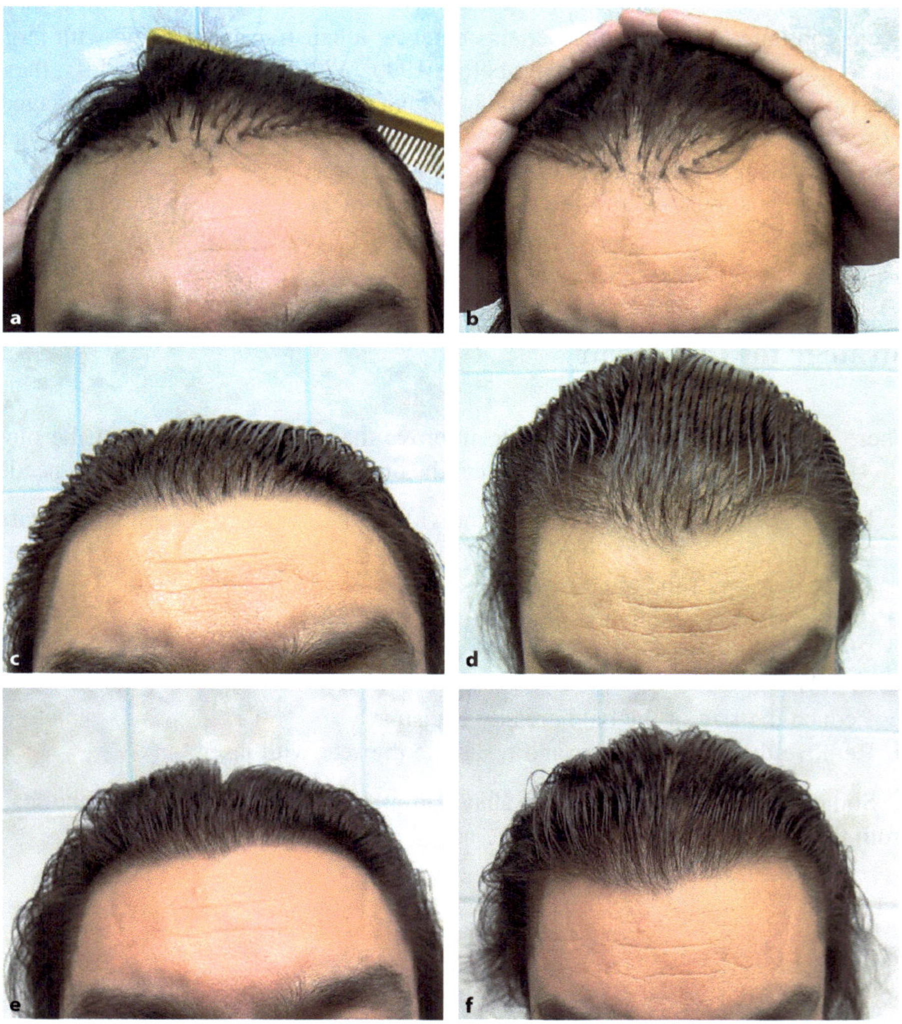

Fig. 1. **a** Preoperative view (1). **b** Preoperative view (2). **c** One year postoperative (1). **d** One year postoperative (2). **e** After second session (1). **f** After second session (2). **a**, **b** Preoperative. **c**, **d** One year postoperative after 1576 follicular unit grafts. **e**, **f** One year postoperative after second session of 1765 grafts

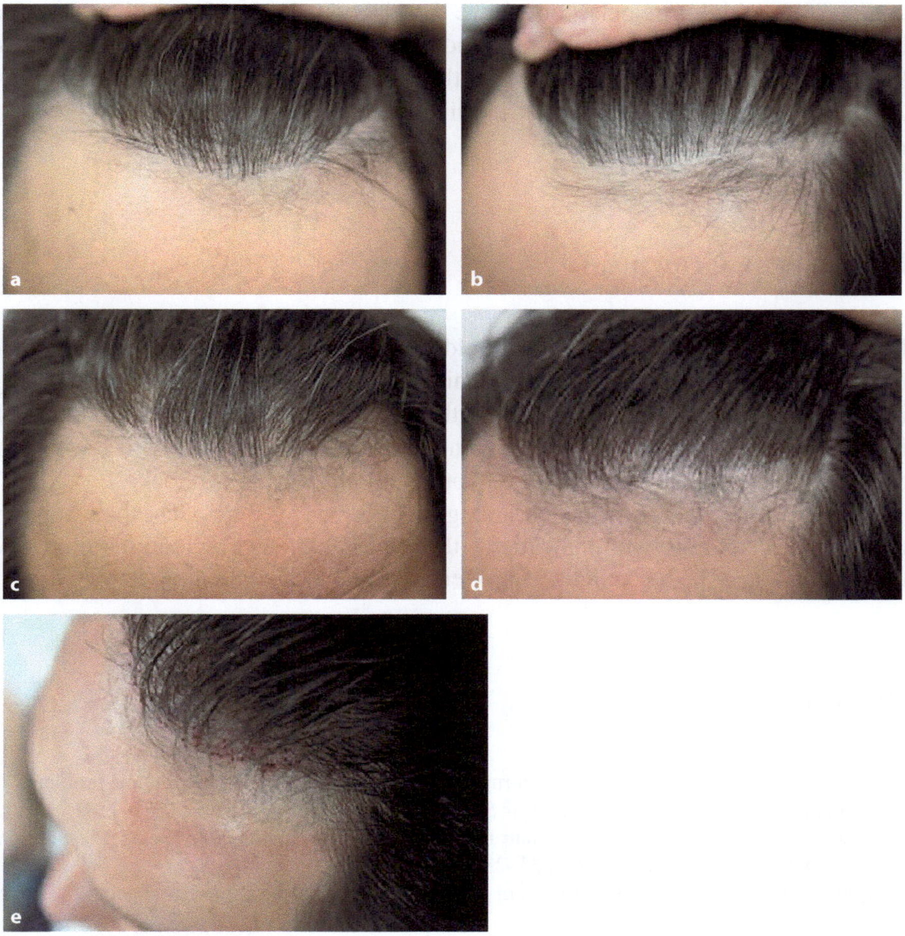

Fig. 2. **a**, **b** Preoperative; **c**, **d** postoperative. **e** Partial removal of mini-grafts by follicular unit extraction (FUE) (courtesy of K. Imagawa)

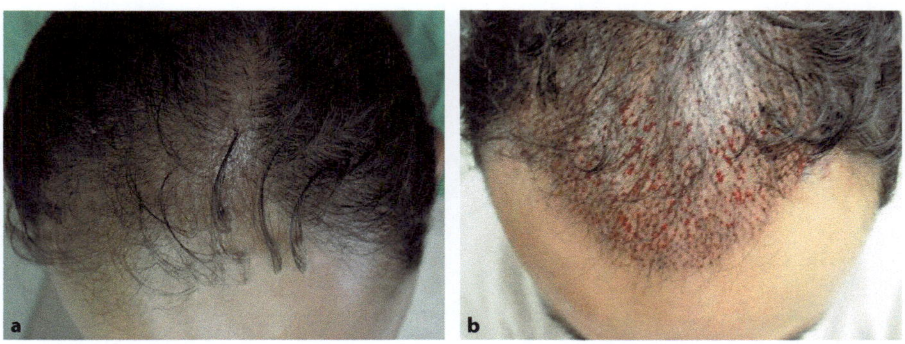

Fig. 3. **a** Preoperative (courtesy of Dr. J.C. Kim). **b** Immediately postoperative

and recreate a high forelock 8 cm above the glabella. The grafts are then recycled by dissecting into follicular unit grafts and transplanted. However, the patients must be informed that scars will be left in the forehead upon removal of the plugs. Alternatively, hair along the lower hairline can be removed by laser followed by resurfacing the scars.

Plugs at the Crown

Plugs at the center of the crown should all be removed and recycled as single follicular unit grafts, bearing in mind hair loss is progressive. If the donor supply is limited and the baldness is extensive, the creation of an isolated frontal forelock is an alternative. However, the intention must first be discussed with the patient as most Asian patients would not be happy with an isolated forelock.

In conclusion, there are many strategies in repairing plugs. The hair surgeon must discuss carefully with the patients that many sessions might be required, and the outcome may be a cosmetic improvement to a certain extent.

References

1. Vogel JE (2000) Correction of the cornrow hair transplant and other common problems in surgical hair restoration. Plast Reconstr Surg 105:1528–1536; discussion 1537–1541
2. Ebstein JS (1999) Revision surgical hair restoration: repair of undesirable results. Plast Reconstr Surg 104:222–232; discussion 233–236
3. Vogel JE (2004) Correcting problems in hair restoration surgery: an update. Facial Plast Surg Clin N Am 12:263–278
4. Unger W (2004) Correction of cosmetic problems in hair transplanting. In: Hair transplantation, 4th edn. Dekker, New York, pp 663–687

Repair of Scalp Flap

K. Imagawa

Unhappy patients after scalp flap surgeries usually have the following kinds of complaints.

Abrupt and Straight Hairline

Fleming and Mayer reported that this problem could be prevented by the same technique used in trichophytic donor closure (see the chapter, Donor Wound Closure by Pathomvanich, this volume) [1]. Nevertheless, I had abandoned this closing technique in the temporo-parieto-occipital (TPO) flap because recurrent folliculitis often occurred. This complication may be a result of the Asian forehead skin being thick and oily as the technique is commonly employed with Caucasians.

Hair transplantation provides the best solution for this complaint. During the repair procedure, it is important to create micro-irregularities along the frontal hairline. Grafts should also be placed around the temporal hairline to camouflage the edge of the flap. Here slits should be made in a way that matches the angle and direction of the flap hair (Fig. 1a,b).

Hair Loss in the Scalp Flap

This condition is either caused by total or partial necrosis in the scalp flap that had not been treated carefully or because the scalp flap was taken from an area that was at risk of later hair loss. Both are good indications for hair transplantation (Fig. 2).

Hair Loss in the Areas from Which the Scalp Flap Was Taken

This is a common complaint, resulting from insufficient undermining and excessive tension on closure. The technique of repair is the same as for hair transplantation in other scar tissue (see the chapter, Repair of Iatrogenic Scarring and Non-Scarring Alopecia from Cosmetic Surgery by Pathomvanich, this volume) (Fig. 3a,b).

D. Pathomvanich and K. Imagawa (eds.), *Hair Restoration Surgery in Asians*
DOI 10.1007/978-4-431-99659-0_39, © Springer 2010

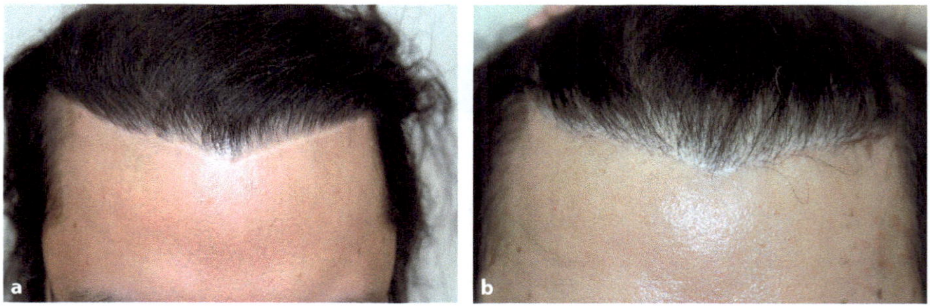

Fig. 1. Abrupt and straight hairline. **a** Patient underwent bilateral temporoparietal flaps by another surgeon in the 1990s. **b** View 18 months after second session of follicular unit transplantation (FUT) (total, 450 grafts)

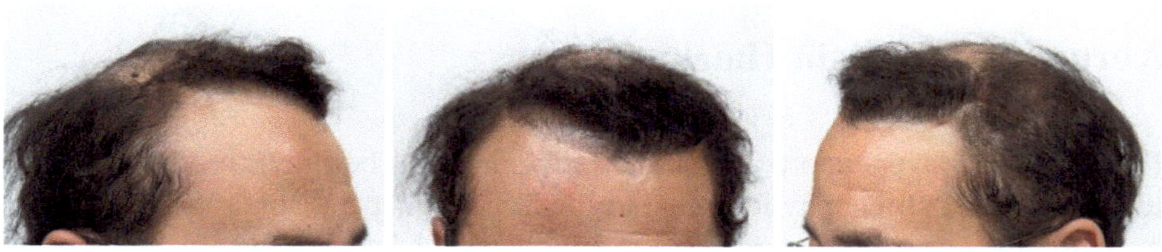

Fig. 2. Hair loss in the flap. Patient underwent bilateral temporoparietal flaps by another surgeon in the late 1990s. Right flap was taken from balding area and started to go bald

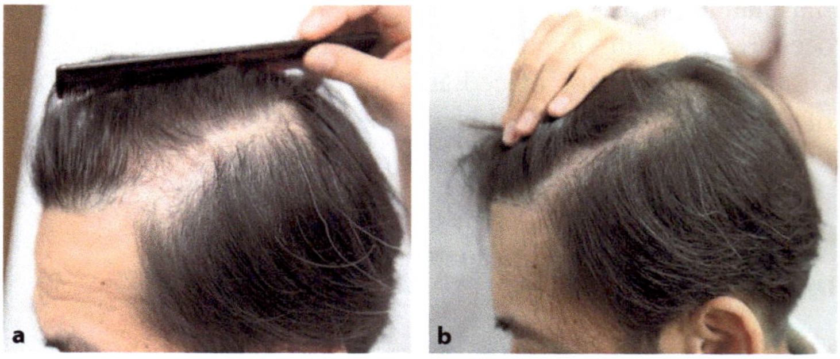

Fig. 3. Hair loss in the area from where flap was taken. **a** Patient underwent temporo-parieto-occipital (TPO) flap by another surgeon in the 1990s. **b** At 12 months after one session of FUT (460 grafts)

Progressive Hair Loss Behind the Scalp Flap

As male pattern hair loss/female pattern hair loss (MPHL/FPHL) progresses, many patients will suffer further loss of hair in the area behind the scalp flap. If hair transplantation is planned, a large number of donor hairs will be required for the thinning area, and it is usually impractical to attempt to match the high density of the scalp flap (Fig. 4a,b).

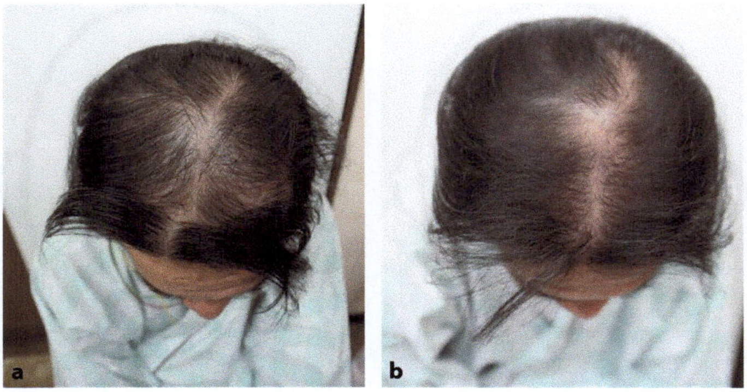

Fig. 4. Hair loss behind TPO flap. **a** Patient underwent temporo-parieto-occipital (TPO) flap by another surgeon in the 1990s. **b** At 12 months after one session of FUT (1100 grafts)

Too-Thick Appearance of the Scalp Flap

Brandy reported a technique for lowering the density of a scalp flap by using a punch 2–3 mm in diameter to extract follicles from the front edge [2]. The author prefers a 1.0- to 1.2-mm punch to remove the grafts under 3× to 4× magnification, and then to recycle the follicles after proper trimming.

Patients should be advised that several sessions may be required and each time the flap has to be shaved.

Poor Hairline Design with Blunt Frontotemporal Angle

Extremely unnatural and apelike hairlines caused by bad location of the flap are described in Western literature, but fortunately this complaint is not common in Asians, possibly because of the Asian anatomical hairline features. The author thinks that the wide frontotemporal angle and straight hairline of Asians might conceal the flappers' poor techniques and make these less conspicuous.

This condition can be repaired in two ways:

1. Incisions are made lateral and posterior to the flap as described by Mayer and Fleming [1] when a dog-ear at the anterior margin of the flap still exists.
2. A fusiform shape of forehead skin is excised anterior to the frontotemporal hairline of the flap as described by Brandy [2] and Beehner [3] (Fig. 5a,b).

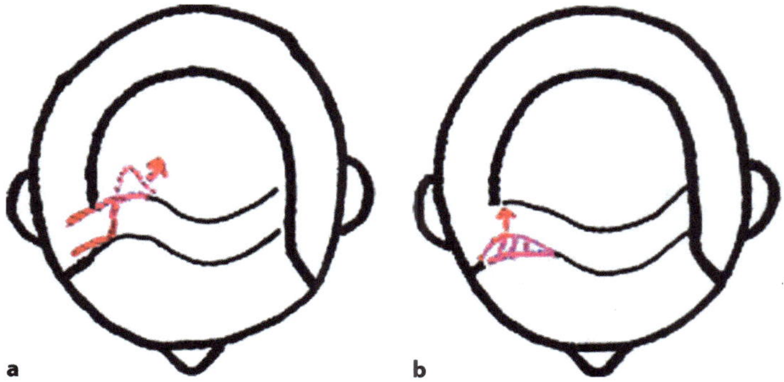

Fig. 5. The repair of blunt frontotemporal angle. **a** Lateral and posterior incision of the flap. **b** Anterior incision of the flap

A Backward Hair Direction

Explanation must be given to the patients that it is almost impossible to change hair direction of the established temporo-parieto-occipital (TPO) and temporoparietal (TP) flap, and in fact such backward hair direction has an advantage in camouflaging hair loss behind the flap. Ohmori of Japan developed a microsurgical free flap to overcome the problem of hair direction from flaps (see the chapter, Advantages of Microvascular Free Scalp Flap Transfer as a Means of Hair Transplantation by Ohmori). Unfortunately, the density of hair within these flaps created difficulties with subsequent hair styling and these flaps never became popular.

It is important to keep in mind that most patients after flap surgery have a tight scalp and overall lower hair density because of extensive undermining and traction. The total number of grafts available for transplantation is therefore limited. These patients very often have several complaints about the flap and their progressing baldness, which cannot all be repaired in a single procedure. Surgery must therefore be planned carefully, the priority of the patient's complaints must be identified, and the number of grafts estimated for each problem. When faced with a limited supply of grafts, it is important to group them into selected areas to achieve satisfactory density. Placing a small number of grafts into a large area will never achieve patient satisfaction.

Don't spread the battlefield!

References

1. Mayer TG, Fleming RW (1992) Aesthetic and reconstructive surgery of the scalp. In: Creation of irregular trichophytic hairline. Mosby Yearbook, St. Louis, pp 121–124
2. Brandy DA (2003) Corrective hair restoration techniques for the aesthetic problems of temporoparietal flaps. Dermatol Surg 29:230–234
3. Beehner ML (1999) Raising a low flap border. Hair Transplant Int 9:118–119

Repair of Artificial Fiber Implantation

K. Imagawa

The U.S. Food and Drug Administration (FDA) has banned the use of artificial hair fiber since 1982. However, other than the United States and Canada, artificial fiber implantation (AI) is permitted as a medical procedure by authorities all over the world. Disputes remain in regard to the frequency and severity of the potential risks of AI.

Some of these complications are as follows:

1. Formation of pits and sebum plug pits where the fiber enters the scalp.
2. Between 20% and 50% of the artificial fibers will gradually fall out each year and have to be replaced to maintain hair density.
3. There are risks of foreign-body reaction, inflammatory reactions, and infections.
4. Over months to years, the artificial fibers tend to migrate short distances in the scalp and clump together into little clusters, looking not unlike small punch-grafts. These are much more likely to become infected than are isolated artificial hairs.
5. Breakage of the fiber can be a problem and is more common in some types of artificial fibers than with others. The Japanese Nido Z-type fiber is very resistant to breakage, but it will still occur with repeated rubbing or scratching by the patient [1].

Complications of AI have been treated mostly by manual removal of fibers and fiber-stubs with forceps and by scalp excisions and scalp flaps in extreme cases. It would be thought that all these patients who have suffered complications would prefer hair transplantation, but this is not always the case. Some prefer to have the troublesome artificial hairs removed and return to the semibald state. Dr. Shiell, in a personal communication with the author in 2008, commented that many others would request the insertion of more artificial fibers once the infection has subsided. The instantaneous nature of artificial hair implantation seems to have much appeal to these patients, and Shiell stated that he found it extremely difficult to convince them of the many advantages of hair transplantation.

When considering repair with hair transplantation, it is very important to first answer two questions during the initial assessment:

D. Pathomvanich and K. Imagawa (eds.), *Hair Restoration Surgery in Asians*
DOI 10.1007/978-4-431-99659-0_40, © Springer 2010

1. Whether infection or inflammation is still active at the recipient scalp.
2. Whether the patient agrees to remove the remaining fibers.

The fibers should be checked for any redness at the point of insertion, which is a sign of infection. The inflammation will usually subside with appropriate antibiotics, but when inflammation or infection is recurrent and persistent, all fibers must be removed. It is important however to obtain the patient's consent to this intervention before proceeding. When there is no sign of infection, it is possible to perform hair transplantation satisfactorily with the artificial fibers in place.

Based on the answers to the two questions, the patient is then categorized into one of three groups.

Group 1: Unhappy Patient Who Has Already Discontinued AI

Remove the remaining fibers followed by hair transplantation in a single-stage procedure; this can be performed when the number of artificial fibers is small. If the number is considerable, the fibers should be removed in advance. The fibers are grasped by artery forceps and pulled very slowly along their exiting directions. The fibers are made of materials such as polybutylene, polyethylene, and nylon with different breakage points, and great care must be excised in removing the fibers lest the fiber breaks off inside the scalp. Punches of 0.75 mm or 1 mm are used to remove those fibers buried deep into the scalp that cannot be reached by the forceps.

After the fibers are removed, the surgeon can proceed immediately to hair transplantation. The overall technique is rather similar to transplanting into scar tissue (see the chapter, Cicatricial Alopecia in Hair Transplantation by Pathomvanich, in this volume) (Fig. 1a,b).

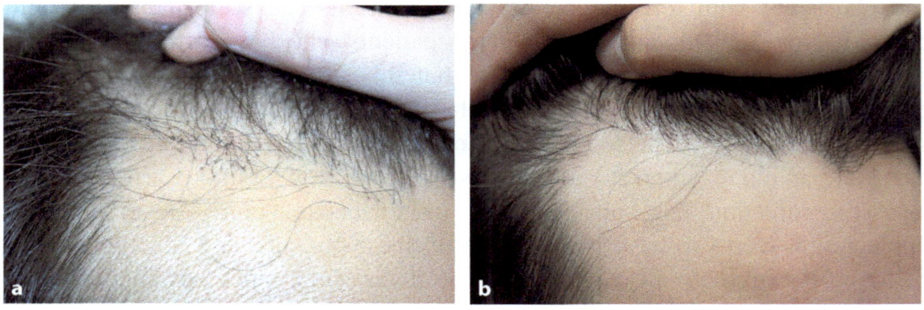

Fig. 1. The repair of a group 1 patient. **a**. A 34-year-old man, Norwood class II. **b** At 2 years after one session of follicular unit transplantation (FUT) (750 grafts)

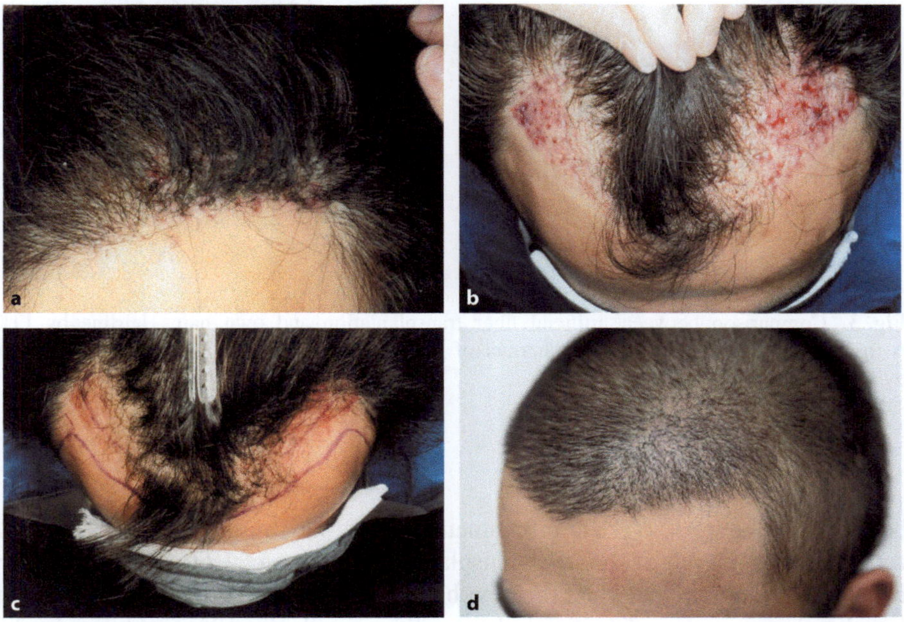

Fig. 2. The repair of a group 2 patient: a 29-year-old man, Norwood class II. **a** Preoperative view of the hairline. **b** Immediately after extraction of the fibers. **c** One month after extraction when the first session of FUT was performed. **d** One year after the third session of FUT (total, 3470 grafts)

Group 2: Patient Who Has Infection from the Fibers

Infection is one potentially serious complication of AI. The only way to control persistent infection is to extract all the fibers. After extraction it may take several months before the infection and inflammation subside completely, and many broken fibers will be missed. Uebel recommended carrying out this second stage of hair transplantation 3 to 4 months after extraction [2].

Obviously all patients want to see their own hairs growing as soon as possible. I believe the second stage can be performed as early as 1 month after extraction so long as there is no clinical sign of infection. I have performed both extraction and hair transplantation as a one-stage procedure and the result was good. Needless to say, I would not recommend this for all cases [3] (Fig. 2a–d).

Group 3: Patients Who Refuse to Remove the Remaining Fibers

Even when there is no infection, placing grafts into areas occupied by a considerable amount of artificial fibers is most likely the worst scenario for hair surgeons

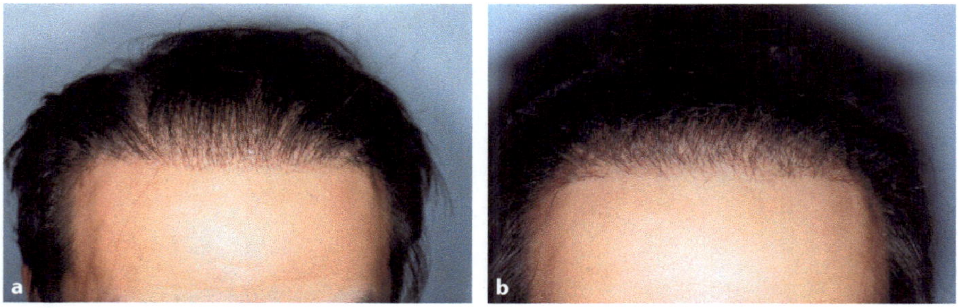

Fig. 3. Comparison between artificial fiber transplantation and own hair. Hairline by FUT is thinner compared with the same amount of fibers. **a** Artificial fiber implantation. **b** Repair by FUT

because any future low-grade inflammation in the nearby artificial hair implants can affect the growth of the new transplants. Furthermore, 10 to 12 months after hair transplantation, and when the new hairs are starting to grow to a meaningful length, a large number of artificial fibers will have fallen out. It would then be difficult for the patient to recognize any increase in the hair volume. As synthetic fibers are generally of larger diameter than human hair, the patient may feel that the hair coverage after hair transplantation is not as good as that from the artificial hair (Fig. 3a,b).

It is possibly better not to accept this group of patients for surgery as the level of satisfaction is usually very low. Alternatively, the patient must be fully informed that an increase in hair volume may not be recognized. A written consent should be obtained before proceeding with transplant surgery.

References

1. Imagawa K (2006) Pros and cons of artificial hair implantation. J Jpn Soc Aesthetic Plast Surg 28:212–218 (in Japanese)
2. Uebel CO (2000) Hair restoration, micrograft & flaps. OESP Grafica S/A, Sao Paulo, pp 307–308
3. Imagawa K (2006) Correction of the complications in artificial hair implantation. J Jpn Soc Aesthetic Plast Surg 28:219–225 (in Japanese)

Part XII
Special Procedures in Hair Restoration Surgery

Eyebrow Transplant

K. Laorwong and D. Pathomvanich

It is generally accepted that dense, wide, and dark-colored eyebrows make the face more charming and attractive in men.

The shape, hair direction, and preference for eyebrows do vary considerably from country to country, even though they may be relatively similar within each particular region. For example, in the Middle East population eyebrows joined in the midline are relatively common and is considered to be a symbol of beauty. On the other hand, this is rather uncommon in the Chinese and Japanese populations and carries a negative impression, while bushy eyebrows are a sign of strength, power, prosperity, and charm in the male.

Overall, there are not many differences between men and women. Obviously, men have wider eyebrows. Most women often pluck or shave the lower border of their eyebrows, especially at the lateral third, to make them more narrow for a more aesthetically pleasing appearance.

The eyebrows remain an important cosmetic asset of the face; some individuals may suffer significant distress on the absence of eyebrows [1]. Eyebrow transplantation is therefore performed to improve the appearance and self-esteem [2].

Indications for Eyebrow Transplantation [3]

1. Congenital absence of eyebrows.
2. Inactive autoimmune diseases such as alopecia areata.
3. Alopecia from infection: for example, TB or leprosy.
4. Defect or loss from tattoo removal using laser or acid; or from trauma such as burn and laceration; or a healed detectable linear scar across the eyebrow from direct brow lift.
5. Enhancement of normal eyebrows by thickening.
6. Uneven eyebrows lacking the lateral third (Queen Anne's sign, which is associated with hypothyroidism) or medial portion of the brow.

Eyebrow reconstructing techniques using micro-grafts of various sizes usually yield good results. Transplanting methods vary from physician to physician. Some

D. Pathomvanich and K. Imagawa (eds.), *Hair Restoration Surgery in Asians*
DOI 10.1007/978-4-431-99659-0_41, © Springer 2010

use 19 G to 21 G needle stick-and-place; some use implanters; while others do premade incisions with a tiny micro-blade such as 15° Sharpoint followed by graft placement.

Many Asian patients who need restoration have patchy or thin and low-density eyebrows. In fact, Asians have less density but coarser-caliber hair, and high skin–hair color contrast, compared to Caucasians. The difference in hair character is the most important reason only single-hair grafts should be used to restore a natural-looking brow. An ultra-skinny single-hair graft should be meticulously dissected under a 10× stereomicroscope to ensure only single hairs will grow. Stick-and-place insertion using a 23 or 24 G needle and under 3× loupe magnification improve the outcome by increasing density and matching the graft size with needle size. The success of reconstruction depends on the surgeon's knowledge of eyebrow anatomy and the ability to reproduce the angle and direction of single hair grafts to achieve a natural result.

Anatomy of the Eyebrow

Eyebrow transplantation is not a commonly performed procedure compared to scalp hair transplantation. Knowledge of eyebrow anatomy and hair direction is essential in achieving a satisfactory result.

We have randomly examined the eyebrows of a total of 20 normal men and women of Thai origin. Recruiting a larger sample was not deemed necessary as the measurements were almost identical. We believe some people of other ethnic groups would share similar features. The results are as follows.

Shape: like a sword with a linear base. The upper part bowed with a pointed tail. The medial and distal ends lie on essentially the same horizontal line except in younger individuals in whom the lateral end is slightly higher. With aging, the entire brow sags downward with the lateral segment generally lower than the medial end.

Size: The average distance between the medial brows was 2.3 cm in both men and women. The average lengths of an eyebrow were 5.5 and 5.0 cm, and the maximum width 1.5 cm and 1.3 cm, in men and women, respectively.

Positioning: The end of a medial brow measured 6 mm in men and 5 mm in women located just below the orbital rim medial to medial canthus (Fig. 1). The highest point of the brow, which appears like the top of a roof, is about 1 cm above the orbital rim between the lateral limbus and the lateral canthus. The tail of the brow is situated lateral to the superolateral orbital rim in the same horizontal plane as the medial brow. In short, the entire brow in Asians is above the orbital rim in contrast with Caucasians where it is located just below the orbital rim.

Hair characters: At its most medial end, the hairs are of small caliber, lighter in color, and point upward for a half centimeter, then point upward and laterally with an increase in diameter. Once approaching the midportion, the hairs in the

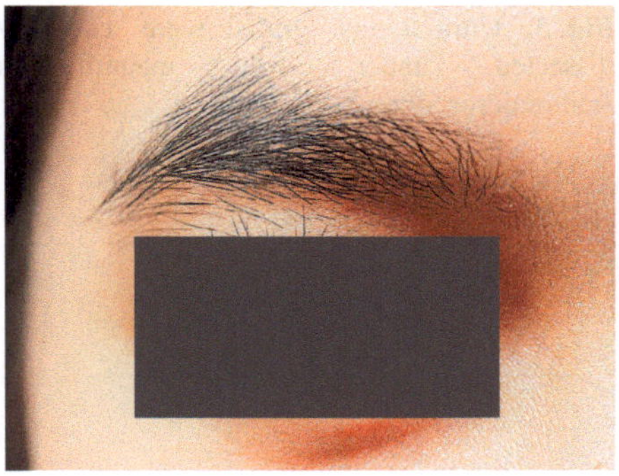

Fig. 1. Normal eyebrow in a Thai female

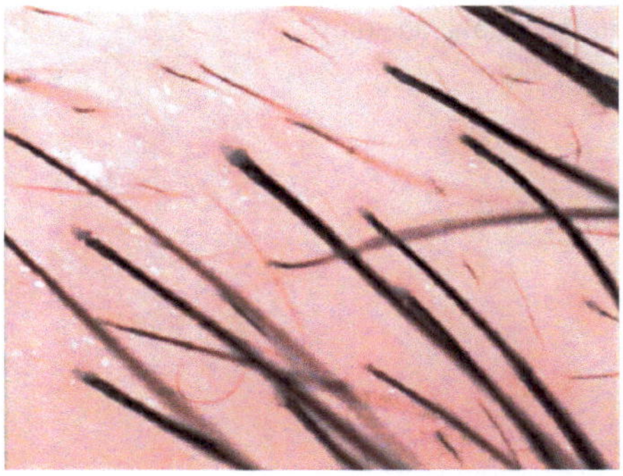

Fig. 2. Eyebrow hairs under 30× magnification microscope are single-hair follicles in both genders

upper and lower portion flow toward each other with a central convergence until the end of the tail. However, there are variances in some individuals in that the hairs only point downward. The hairs exit at a more acute angle, but their small caliber and the short pointed ends create an illusion of flat angle. Central convergence begins at the medial limbus. The brow at the middle third is wider and denser. Once approaching the tail, the hairs have a smaller caliber and lesser density [4]. Follicular units of an eyebrow were examined using a digital USB microscope (Scalar) and found to contain only single hairs in both genders under 30× magnification (Fig. 2.)

Surgical Techniques

The surgeon and patient should agree in the outline of the eyebrow and mark it in the sitting position. Matching the size of existing eyebrow with donor hair is done with micro-caliber whenever possible. The donor site is selected from the mid-occipital area to match the caliber of the existing brow (it is least likely to turn gray). The number of grafts depends on the size and feature of the intended

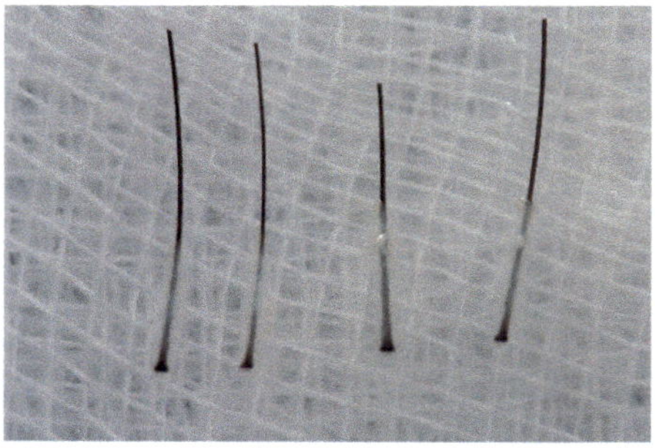

Fig. 3. Ultra-skinny grafts were carefully dissected under 10× magnification stereomicroscope

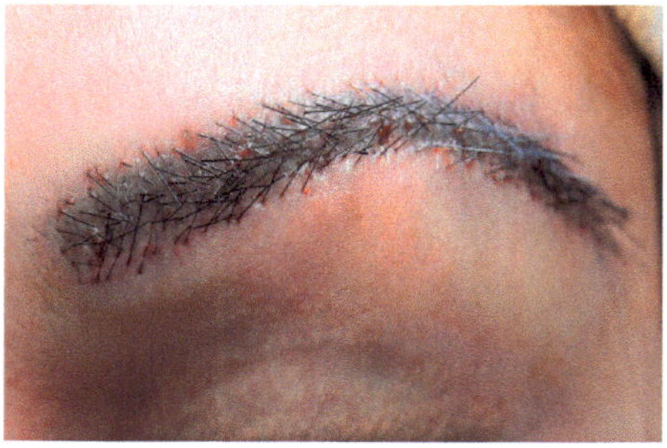

Fig. 4. Direction in the medial third will be parallel to the brow axis instead of upward as in the normal anatomy

reconstruction of the brow. On average, 100 to 300 single-hair grafts are required on each side. The donor hairs are trimmed to 1 cm long.

We use routinely the open harvesting technique [5] and 3× magnifying loupes to harvest donor hair. The wound is closed with trichophytic technique (de-epithelizing the lower edge) and in a single layer using absorbable sutures.

The single-hair grafts are carefully dissected under 10× microscopic magnification (Fig. 3). Ultra-skinny single follicular unit grafts can be produced by trimming away the surrounding fat and tissue, leaving behind the outer root sheath. Follicular units that contain two hairs or more are longitudinally sectioned into one-hair units.

The brow area is cleansed with betadine and anesthetized with 1% xylocaine with epinephrine; no tumescent fluid is required. A 3× loupe magnification is preferred to perform simultaneous stick-and-place; 23 G and sometimes 24 or 25 G needles can be used for flat angle insertion and dense packing. This technique can easily be mastered after training.

When inserting the grafts it is important to align the hair shaft with the axis of the brow; otherwise, the hair will flow out of the axis, resulting in an unnatural look. For uniform density and symmetry, the eyebrow is divided into three portions. One should first determine how many grafts are to be placed in each segment. In a normal individual, hairs in the superior margin of the medial third direct upward and away from the brow axis. The transplanted hair should instead direct downward and flow along the brow axis (Fig. 4). This modification is necessary because the transplanted hairs are thicker and when inserted in an upward direction in the medial region may produce unnatural growth [1]. For the middle and lateral portions, the hairs should converge to each other. Here the needle is inserted in an almost flat angle (Fig. 5). For the lateral segment, the border is feathered superiorly and inferiorly, and a lesser density is usually adequate (Fig. 5). Overall, the borders of the eyebrow must be irregular with finer-caliber hairs transplanted in the peripheral area. Before completion, the patient should examine the transplanted eyebrows and adjustment be made accordingly (Figs. 6, 7, 8).

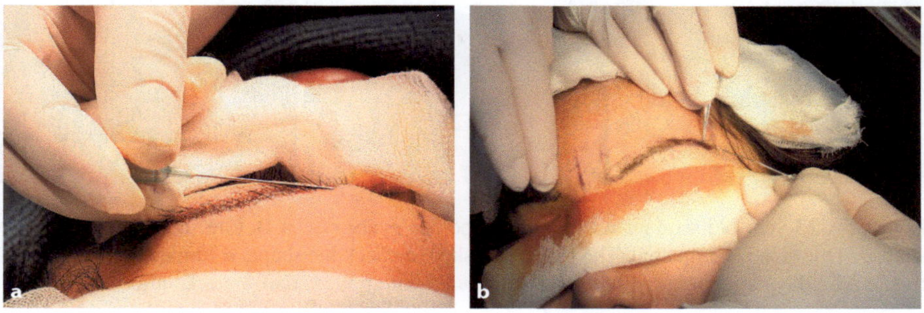

Fig. 5. **a** The needle is inserted in at acute angle to be almost flat to the skin. **b** Direction and angle are crucial in planting the tail

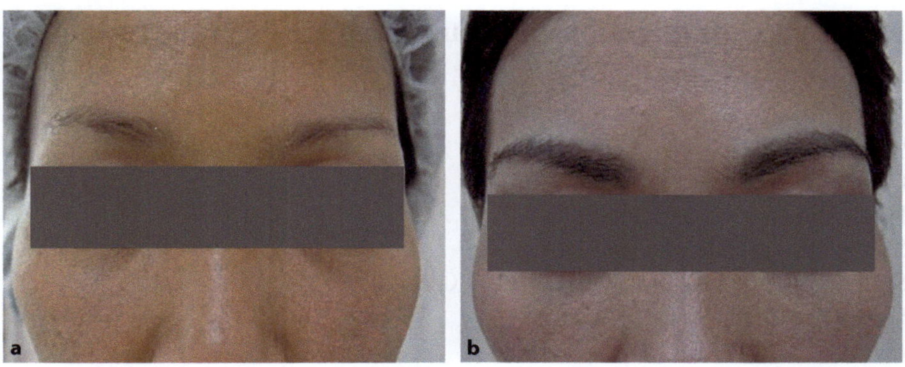

Fig. 6. **a** Eyebrows in female with thinning eyebrow (before). **b** At 6 months after 425 grafts

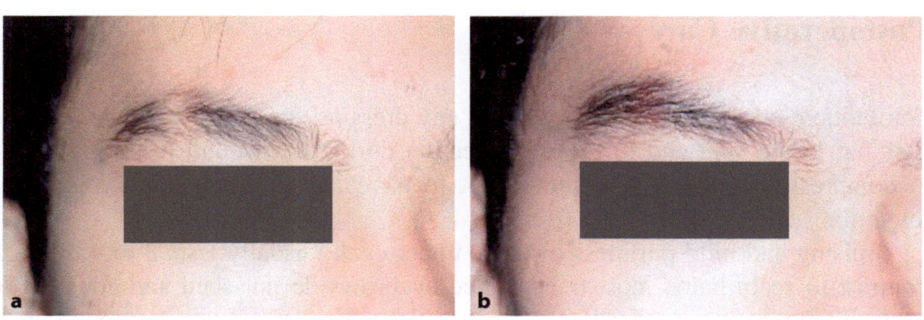

Fig. 7. **a** Scar in eyebrow. **b** After hair transplantation

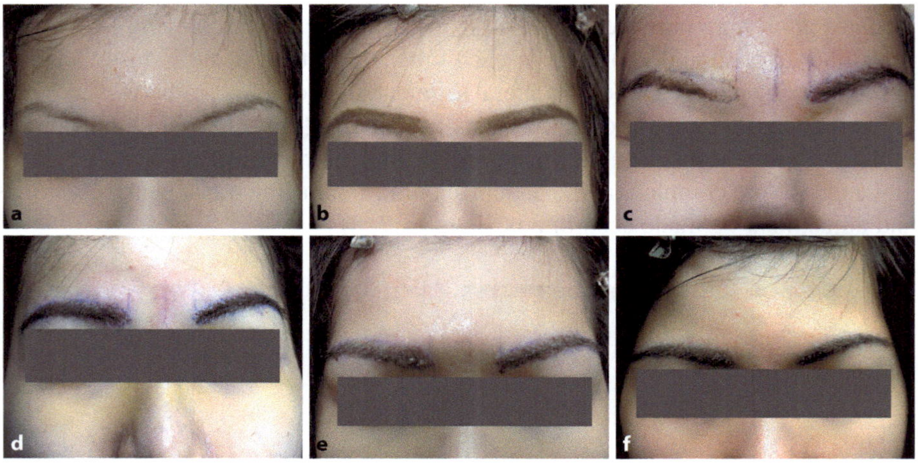

Fig. 8. A 23-year-old woman wants to reshape her eyebrows. **a** Before. **b** Outline of desired shape. **c** One side is completed. The patient is asked to check the shape. **d** Immediately postoperative. **e** At 2 days after surgery, with antibiotic ointment applied. **f** At 2 weeks after surgery

Keys and Considerations in Transplanting Asian Eyebrows

Anatomy and character of eyebrows
Single-hair unit
Coarse hair caliber
High skin–hair color contrast
Skinny single follicular unit hair graft
Stick-and-place insertion with 23 or 24 G needles
Dense packing
Flat angle insertion

Postoperative Care

Antibiotic eye ointment is used without any dressing for 10 days to maintain the hair flat to the skin and to prevent infection during the wound healing process. A compressed dressing was shown not to have any advantage in keeping the angle flat.

Bruising and mild puffiness over the upper eyelid usually lasts 3 to 4 days. In contrast to scalp hairs, most transplanted eyebrows do not shed and continue to grow. Trimming once a week is required. If the patient requires any touch-up in density, a time frame of at least 6 months is recommended.

Complications

1. Improper hair direction and asymmetrical appearance of the eyebrows are the most common complaints encountered.
2. Folliculitis rarely occurs.
3. Bruising and swelling are common but self-limiting except in an unusual bleeder.
4. Hypertrophic scar and keloid have not been encountered.
5. Pitting and ingrown hair are also not seen.

References

1. Kim JC, Choi YC (1996) Hair transplantation of eyelashes and eyebrows. In: Stough DB, Haber RS (eds) Hair replacement: surgical and medical. Mosby, St. Louis, pp 261–268
2. Goldwyn RM (1991) The patient and plastic surgeon. Little, Brown, Boston, p 52
3. Gandelman IM (1983) Patient selection in hair transplantation. Annals of Brazilian Symposium on Facial Contour, Sao Paulo, Brazil
4. Pathomvanich D (2004) Anatomical restoration surgery of the eyebrow in Asian. Thai J Surg 25:47–52
5. Pathomvanich D (2000) Donor harvesting: a new approach to minimize transection of hair follicles. Dermtol Surg 26:345–348
6. Pouteaux P (1993) How to survive with difficult patients. Presented at The International Society of Hair Surgeons World Congress Meeting, Dallas, TX, April 1993
7. Nordstram REA (1977) Eyebrow reconstruction by punch hair transplantation. Plast Reconstr Surg 60:74–76
8. Nordstram REA (1988) Eyebrow reconstruction with small free grafts of scalp. In: Unger WP, Nordstram REA (eds) Hair transplantation, 2nd edn. Dekker, New York, pp 310–316
9. Vallis CP (1982) Hair transplantation for the treatment of male pattern baldness. Thomas, Springfield, pp 392–406
10. Gandelman M (1995) Eyebrow and eyelash transplantation. In: Unger WP (ed) Hair transplantation, 3rd edn. Dekker, New York, pp 294–306
11. Kim JC, Choi YC (2004) Eyebrow, eyelash, mustache, and pubic area hair transplantation. In: Unger WP, Shapiro R (eds) Hair transplantation, 4th edn. Dekker, New York, pp 579–580
12. Arakawa I (1967) Cosmetic evaluation of eyebrow surgery with transplants of single hairs. Jpn J Plast Reconstr Surg 10:1
13. Ishiko S (1965) Repair of eyebrow: single hair transplantation, using Kanazashni's needle. Jpn J Plast Reconstr Surg 8:11
14. Tamura H (1943) Pubic hair transplantation. Jpn J Dermatol 53:76
15. Krusius FF (1914) Ueber die Einpflanzung lebender Haare zur Wimpernbildung. Dtsch Med Wochenschr 19:958
16. Marritt E (1980) Transplantation of single hair from the scalp as eyelashes. J Dermatol Surg Oncol 6:271–273
17. Epstein S (2006) Jeffrey eyebrow transplantation. Hair Transplant Forum 16(4), pp 121–123
18. Ergun SS, Sahinoglu K (2003) Eyebrow transplantation. Ann Plast Surg 51:584–586
19. Goldman GD (2001) Eyebrow transplantation. Dermatol Surg 27:352–354
20. Wang J, Fan J (2004) Cicatricial eyebrow reconstruction with a dense-packing one- to two-hair grafting technique. Plast Reconstr Surg 114:1420–1426

Eyelash Transplant

K. Imagawa

Eyelash transplantation is classified into two categories:

1. Reconstructive eyelash transplantation for correction of loss caused by injury, diseases, iatrogenic alopecia, congenital atrichia, or trichotillomania.
2. Aesthetic eyelash transplantation.

Strip graft and pedicle flap [1] are now rarely used for aesthetic eyelash transplantation. The following techniques have been reported and are still in use for both categories:

- Follicular units and reverse follicular units grafting [2,3].
- Double follicular unit grafting [4].
- Single-hair micro-grafting using the "sewing" technique [5] or the Choi/KNU implanter [6].
- Single-hair micro-grafting using eyebrow hair [7].

In East Asia, the use of the Choi/KNU implanter is the standard method (see the chapter by Kim, this volume). The single-hair micro-grafting technique using a 21 or 22 G hypodermic needle, on the other hand, is mentioned more often in Western countries and is described below.

My Method

Eyelash transplantation is performed under mild sedation, and 1% lidocaine with 1 : 100 000 epinephrine is usually used as the local anesthetic solution. The donor site is selected from the occiput or above the ear depending on the individual hair characters, and donor hair is clipped to 1 cm in length.

Follicular unit extraction (FUE) or stripping can also be employed in harvesting donor hair. Eyebrows are not recommended as the donor source because any scarring is likely to be visible in these exposed areas.

After single-hair grafts are obtained under microscopic dissection, 21 or 22 G needles bent by a needle holder are used to create recipient tunnels along the

D. Pathomvanich and K. Imagawa (eds.), *Hair Restoration Surgery in Asians*
DOI 10.1007/978-4-431-99659-0_42, © Springer 2010

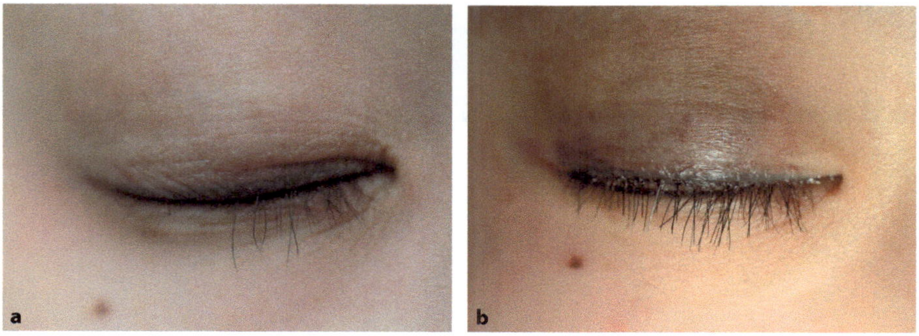

Fig. 1. Reconstructive eyelash transplantation. **a** Before. Patient lost right lashes by laser treatment. **b** Immediately after the procedure

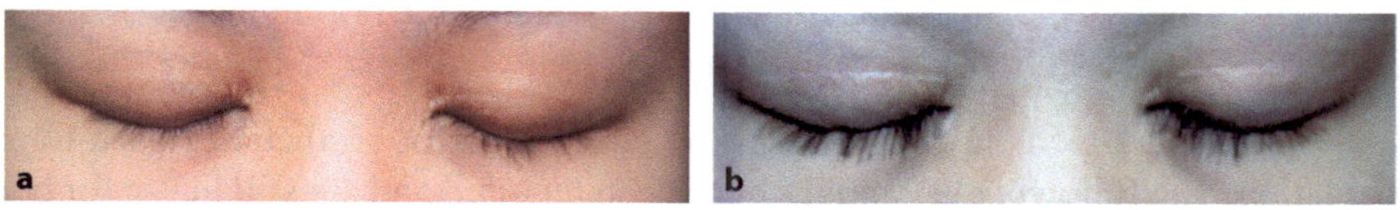

Fig. 2. Aesthetic eyelash transplantation. **a** Before. **b** After

eyelids. Grafts are then inserted carefully using fine jeweler's forceps. Implantation should be done in one or two rows along the eyelids in a curved and fan-shaped manner. A two-step approach is the key to prevent pop-up and increase the number of grafts inserted. First the grafts are inserted on every alternative slit, skipping one in between. On the second round, the skipped slits are filled. Corneal shields are not used during our procedure (Figs. 1, 2). Normally the number of eyelashes on each side is 100 hairs in the upper lid and 60 hairs in the lower lid. The number of transplanted donor hairs per eyelid has been reported as between 20 and 60, and we transplant on average 40 in each upper eyelid. We transplant in the lower eyelid only in case of reconstruction because of the greater difficulty of making appropriate angled pockets.

Although this technique is more time consuming and backbreaking, there are many potential advantages:

- The needle is very cheap and the procedure inexpensive.
- The bent needle can make a more acute angle.
- The bent needle can make a curved pocket.

The bent needle can also be helpful in creating slits in eyebrow, temporal hairline, and sideburn reconstruction. The bevel of the needle should be inserted at a very acute angle when working on the hairline and sideburns (Fig. 3).

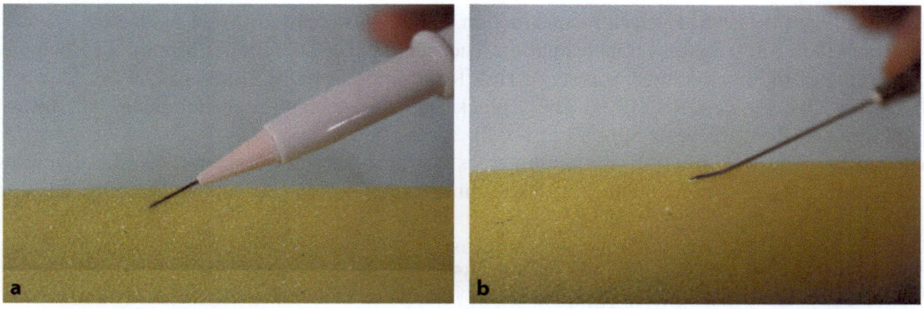

Fig. 3. Comparison between implanter (**a**) and bent hypodermic needle (**b**). The needle can make a very acute angled and curved slit

Postoperative Phase

Donor hair is trimmed to the same length as the original eyelash. A bandage is usually not required. The patient should avoid rubbing the eyes for 24 h after the procedure and use eyeshields while sleeping. Mequitazine 3 mg (antihistaminergic drug) is prescribed to stop itchiness at bedtime when needed. The patient must be informed that transplanted eyelashes would grow like scalp hair and require regular trimming. Curvature can be maintained by using mascara and a curling device. There have been no study of the final survival rate of single-hair micro-grafts in eyelashes, but the author presumes around 80% of the grafts could be expected to come out, and an additional session could be performed 6 months postoperatively by request.

Complications

- The bruising and swelling last 1–2 weeks after surgery in most cases.
- It is rather common to dislodge the grafts if the patient scratches his/her itchy eyelids.
- Tenting may occur because of too superficial graft insertion or pop-up.
- Infection and entropion can occur but are rare.

References

1. Millard DR (1986) Row strip for lashes. In: Principles of plastic surgery. Little, Brown, Boston, p 212
2. Breeling JL (2007) Eyelash transplantation: who, why, and how. Hair Transplant Forum Int 17:17–20

3. Gandelman M (1996) Eyelash reconstruction. Hair Transplant Forum Int 6:18–19
4. Straub PM (2007) Eyelash transplantation. The technique of Dr. Jennifer Martinik. 15th annual meeting of the International Society of Hair Restoration Surgery, Las Vegas, NV
5. Caputy GG, Flowers RS (1994) The " pluck and sew" technique of individual hair follicle placement. Plast Reconstr Surg 93:615–620
6. Choi YC, Kim JC (2004) Transplanting areas that need special consideration. 15A. Eyebrow, eyelash, mustache, and pubic area hair transplantation. In: Hair transplantation, 4th edn. Dekker, New York, pp 579–584
7. Jazayeri K (2008) Eyelash transplantation using eyebrow-derived single-hair grafts: a case report. Hair Transplant Forum Int 18:134–135

Sideburn Transplant

D. Pathomvanich

What Is a Sideburn?

The sideburn is the pre-auricular facial hair that extends to join the temple hair. Gaps in between or failure to join appears esthetically unpleasing. The wide and flared sideburns of Elvis Presley have been popular among men from the mid-1960s until the recent trend to short hairstyles.

On average, South East Asians have minimal or absent sideburns. Because most men cut their hair and sideburns very short, the number of requests for sideburn transplant is quite low, except for the repair of facelift scarring. No doubt such requests will increase if long hair becomes fashionable again.

Sideburn hair, being facial hair, exhibits no pattern baldness, but its distribution varies with race and ethnicity. One should have an idea in regard to its optimal length and width, however, when considering sideburn reconstruction.

The author examined 20 normal Asian men and women in his office. On average, the sideburn was about 1.5 cm in width. It extended from the temple inferiorly to end at the tragus in most cases. It was not common to see sideburns connecting with the beard and mustache, as it frequently does in Caucasians. The posterior hairline of the sideburn was about 2 cm away from the tragal rim. The density was low and with a mixture of one or two hair follicles. Hair texture varied from very coarse to fine hair. Asian men with moderate facial hair and mustache usually have longer and wider sideburns.

Indication for Sideburn Transplant

1. Absent or inadequate sideburn
2. Lost of sideburn from rhytidectomy
3. Scarring alopecia from injury, e.g., burn

The majority of patients seeking sideburn reconstruction are those who have undergone rhytidectomy [1–3]. They usually have an idea of what they want regarding the shape, length, and density of the new sideburn.

D. Pathomvanich and K. Imagawa (eds.), *Hair Restoration Surgery in Asians*
DOI 10.1007/978-4-431-99659-0_43, © Springer 2010

The Procedure

One has to discuss their expectations with the patients before surgery. It is a good idea to paste small pieces of a hairpiece onto the sideburn to visualize the possible end result. The patients can compare difference in density and texture to have an idea what they want. The shape of the sideburn is then drawn to their satisfaction.

The area is calculated by measuring the length and width in centimeters. Density of at least 40–50 follicles/cm^2 is required in men, with a lesser density of 20–30/cm^2 in women. This number is usually adequate to achieve a good look even after a single session.

After knowing the surface area and the desired density, the total number of grafts and thus the size of donor strip can be calculated [4]. (Please refer to the chapter on calculating the donor strip.)

The donor site is selected to match texture with the temple hair, which in return matches well with the sideburn. Hair should be trimmed to 1 cm long before harvesting. One can also use follicular unit extraction (FUE) to extract grafts directly from the temples if the density is adequate.

Local anesthetic containing 1% lidocaine and epinephrine is injected to the entire area intradermally as a ring block. No tumescent fluid is needed because bleeding is usually minimal. Needles (20 G) are used to create premade incisions or to stick-and-place two hair grafts into the middle of the sideburn. In a similar fashion, 21 G needles are used to place single hair grafts along the anterior and posterior borders, and feathering at the end for a natural look. One can also use micro-blades and lateral slits, as described by Hasson and Wong [5].

In women, the end of the sideburn should tail off in a pointed fashion. In men, the end is broader with the hair directing inferiorly at an acute angle.

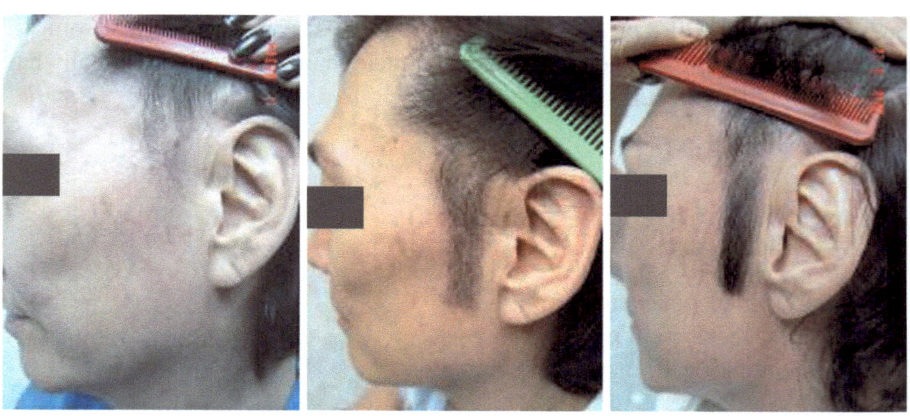

Fig. 1. Creating a new sideburn. *Left*, 2005. *Center*, 16 days after surgery. *Right*, 1 year after surgery

Postoperative Care

After the procedure is completed, the recipient site should be covered with antibiotic ointment followed by nonadhesive dressing. The patients return to the clinic the next day for wound care. A dressing for the first few days is recommended to prevent graft dislodgement in case the patient inadvertently sleeps on that side. The postoperative course is rather simple, but the patient must be careful in washing the face for a week. After that, the grafts should be well adhered. Most of the graft hairs do not shed but continue to grow.

For older patients who may be considering a facelift, the surgeon should advise that a sideburn should be transplanted after the rhytidectomy has been performed. Otherwise, any preexisting sideburn will be pulled towards the ear with an unnatural look.

References

1. Nordstrom REA (1991) Sideburn reconstruction. Plast Reconstruct Surg 88:1107
2. Gandleman M, Epstein J (2004) Hair transplantation to eyebrow, eyelash and other part of the body. Facial Plast Clin N Am 12:253–261
3. Alfonso B (1999) Prevention and correction of the temporal hair loss in rhytidectomy. Plastic Reconst Surg 104:2226–2228
4. Chang S (2001) Estimate number of graft and donor area. Hair Transplant Forum Int 4:97–102
5. Hasson V, Wong J (2002) Coronal recipient sites. Presented at the 10th annual meeting of the International Society of Hair Restoration Surgery in Chicago, IL, October 12

Mustache Transplant

D. Pathomvanich

Mustache transplantation is not as common as eyebrow transplantation. Harris [1], in his recent survey, reported that mustache transplants accounted for only 1% to 1.5% of all hair restoration procedures in 2006. Okuda, from Japan, may be the first physician reporting mustache transplant back in 1939 [2, 6]. The majority of Orientals do not have as much mustache as do their Caucasian and Indian counterparts. Still, there is a steady demand for this facial hair transplant, including beard and goatee.

Reasons for such requests include these:

1. To fill in areas without any beard and mustache to create a new look
2. To increase density in area with existing beard or mustache
3. To camouflage scarring alopecia from accidental or iatrogenic trauma such as repair of cleft lip [5] or tumor excision at the lip

Characteristics of the Mustache

The mustache contains mostly single hairs, and the density varies among different ethnic groups, being higher in those of Indian or Middle East origin and Caucasians. The most obvious difference between mustache and scalp hair is the coarseness of the former. Matching transplanted hair with existing mustache is difficult yet crucial if an unnatural or uneven look is to be avoided. The donor site should be searched carefully for hair of comparable caliber. If the discrepancy cannot be matched, two-hair follicles should be used instead of single-hair grafts to blend in with the existing mustache.

Design

The shape of the mustache is first outlined while the patient is sitting. On approval, it is traced with a marker, and symmetry must be ensured, especially in a goatee.

D. Pathomvanich and K. Imagawa (eds.), *Hair Restoration Surgery in Asians*
DOI 10.1007/978-4-431-99659-0_44, © Springer 2010

It is advisable to transplant beyond the marked area and with a higher density at the center. Dissatisfaction usually arises from inadequate density and a too-narrow goatee, necessitating more sessions. Any excessive or unwanted hair can be simply trimmed short or shaved off. For most Asians, 40 grafts/cm^2 should be adequate. In those who desire very dense coverage, up to 60 grafts/cm^2 may be needed.

Donor Harvesting

The donor area is examined for areas with the coarsest hair. In some people this is at the parietal rather than the mid-occipital area. The donor hair is trimmed to leave a hair stump of about 1 cm. Bouhanna [3] and Wolf [4] advocated long hair grafts, but the short hair grafts have more advantages:

- Pop-up is less during insertion
- The transplanted area is easier to clean during the immediate postoperative period
- Any infection can be diagnosed early and treated promptly
- Fewer grafts will be lost on accidental scratching

The length and width of the donor strip are calculated as previously described. Under local anesthetic, the hair-bearing skin is then excised and the wound closed.

Insertion

As local anesthesia for the recipient site, 1% lidocaine with epinephrine is used. Pain is more intense during injection when compared to the scalp as the face is more sensitive. At times infraorbital and mental nerve block are required to ensure there is no pain during insertion.

The grafts are inserted via the stick-and-place method using 20 G needles for the two-hair grafts. Single-hair grafts are inserted at the end for dense packing using 21 or 22 G needles, or mini-blades of different sizes are chosen to match the grafts. The uppermost row at the periphery should consist of only one-hair grafts to look natural. No tumescent fluid is required other than local anesthetic. In case bleeding is above average, a small amount of epinephrine in high concentration can be injected before further insertion. The direction and angle should follow the existing hair. Otherwise the hairs should point inferoposteriorly at an acute angle. As the skin around the lips is mobile and thinner than the scalp, the grafts are prone to pop out during insertion.

Basically the mustache (facial hair) has no well-defined boundary. Those who desire transplantation always express the wish to keep a long mustache. Because hairs are transplanted only at 40 grafts/cm^2, they should converge slightly toward the midline to achieve a dense look at the philtrum.

Postoperative Care

Antibiotic ointment is applied to cover all the grafts. The wound is then dressed with nonadhesive gauze secured with micropore tape. One can opt to leave the site open, but there is always a chance of contamination and dislodgment of grafts from accidental scratching.

Overall, more attention is demanded in postoperative care than in scalp hair transplant as the grafts are placed on areas easily contaminated by saliva and food during eating. As the lips are mobile and prone to graft-popping, the patient must stay on a liquid diet for a few days and sip only through straws. No tooth brushing is allowed. Oral hygiene is maintained by rubbing the teeth and oral cavity with wet sticky gauze at least four to five times a day. About 3 to 5 days after surgery and in the absence of any sign of infection, the patient is allowed to take solid food. Watching comedy movies, chatting, and smiling are all prohibited in the first few days. An oral broad-spectrum antibiotic should be given for at least a week.

Patient should return daily for wound care until there is no further risk of infection. Antibiotic ointment or Vaseline should be applied frequently to seal the grafts from saliva contamination. Follow-up after 6 months is recommended to check if more density is desired.

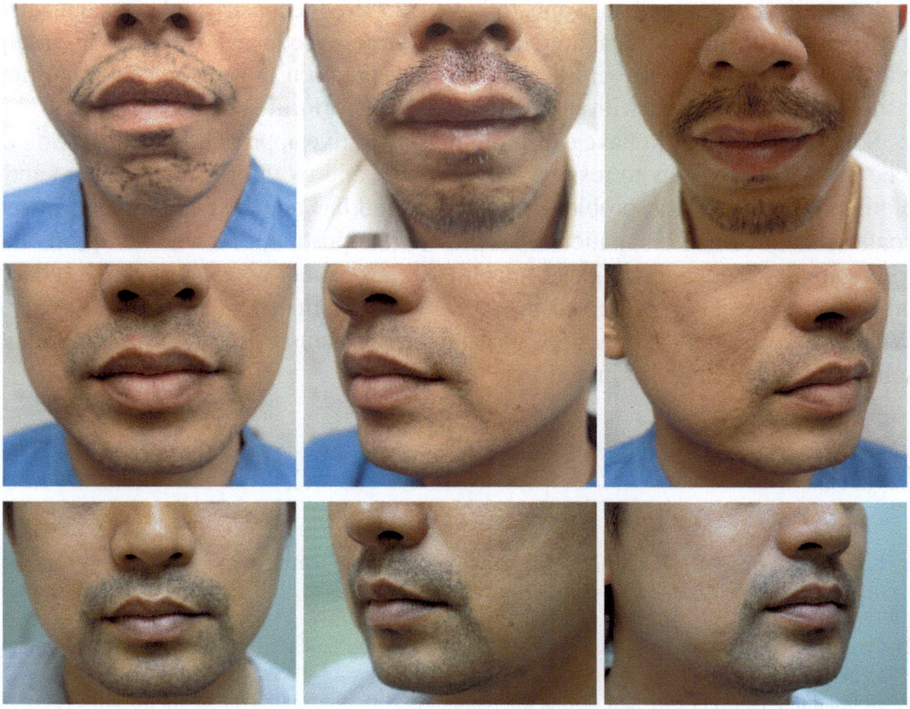

Fig. 1. *Top row, left to right*: Before; immediate postop; after second session in December 2008. *Center row*, before surgery in 2007. *Bottom row*, follow-up after 1 year in 2008

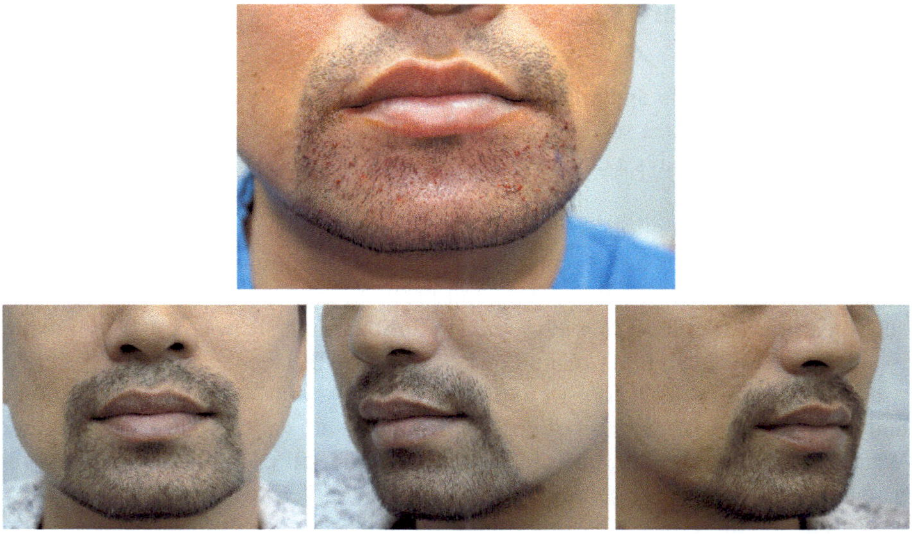

Fig. 2. The three top pictures in Fig. 1 were taken preoperatively in 2007. Patient returned after 1 year to have more grafts fill in the entire chin. *Bottom row*, after second session in December 2008

In cases when the patient wants to have sideburns reconstructed and connected to the mustache and beard, a large number of grafts is required. If he also has scalp hair loss, he may end up with less hair to transplant on the scalp. This important issue must be discussed with the patient to set the priorities before surgery.

Some surgeons might have a different postoperative approach, such as R. Shiell, who allows his patients to resume a normal diet and tooth brushing, uses no antibiotic ointment, with no problem with saliva, and has not seen any infection from contamination. I had one patient with a moderate pustule, one who lost grafts the following day from not being careful, and another patient who had severe infection on day 2; these cases prompted me to be very careful about postoperative care. Whether the differences among Caucasians and Asians in food consumption and self-hygiene contribute to infection is unknown.

References

1. Leonard RT Jr, Sideris K (2007) Survey finds popularity of hair restoration is growing: number of procedures performed worldwide increased 34% since 2004. Hair Transplant Forum 17(4):133
2. Okuda (1939) Clinical and experimental study of living hair transplantation. Jpn J Dermatol Urol 46:6
3. Bouhanna P (2007) Long hair grafts: 20 years of experience. Hair Transplant Forum 17(4):127
4. Wolf BR (2003) Beard and moustache hair transplants. Hair Transplant Forum 13(6)
5. Kolenda M, Kolasinski J (2003) Reconstruction of hair loss of the upper lip in man after plastic operation of the cleft lip and palate. Hair Transplant Forum 13(4)
6. Shiell RC (2004) The Okuda papers. Hair Transplant Forum 14(1)

Chest Hair Transplant

D. Pathomvanich

Some believe that men with chest hair are sexy and more attractive to the opposite sex. Others consider chest hair a nuisance and dislike the ape look. Caucasians, Indians, and people from the Middle East very often have an abundance of chest hair, and many want to have it removed. In contrast, the majority of Orientals do not have chest hair, and some may desire chest hair transplantation to enhance their sexual appeal.

In general, chest hairs, similar to other body hairs, are randomly distributed but most are found in the mid-precordium. The follicle contains a single hair, two hairs, or sometimes three hairs, as found in the scalp. The hair shaft is often curly with an average length of 2–5 cm, usually longer than pubic hair, and with varying direction and angle. Density is low at 20–40 follicles/cm^2. There is a considerable variation in diameter, with an average of 18 μm when compared to the 70 μm that is characteristic of scalp hair [1].

After transplantation there is a potential to lose the grafts with low yield for several reasons:

1. Chest skin is not as thick as scalp skin
2. Body movement involving the chest wall may cause the grafts to pop or sink during the immediate postoperative period
3. Rubbing with clothing or accidentally with other objects
4. Sweating

Patient Selection

The patient must first be evaluated as to whether he has the potential to develop male pattern baldness (MPB). If he has a personal or family history of MPB, the

D. Pathomvanich and K. Imagawa (eds.), *Hair Restoration Surgery in Asians*
DOI 10.1007/978-4-431-99659-0_45,

patient should be warned that the use of donor hair as chest hair will lessen the reserve for future scalp hair transplant should his baldness become progressive. He has to decide what is more important to him. Obviously, without such risk, the decision is easy.

Planning and Procedure

Because the chest area is large, it is crucial to properly design the pattern of the chest hair. The following considerations must be addressed.

1. What kind of shape and hair distribution does the patient desire? Should it be triangular, rhomboidal, or rectangular in shape?
2. How to achieve a sexy, attractive, yet natural look?
3. What density is required to meet the goal?
4. The extent of the transplant: how far one should go toward the neck as well as the umbilicus?
5. Where to obtain the donor hair: the scalp, pubis, body, or axilla?

Most patients will guide the physician in regard to what they want in the design and density. I use scalp hair as the donor site as a large number of grafts can be obtained per strip. Pubic or axillary hair provides an alternative source. Although the yield of these grafts is less when compared to scalp hair, it can create a more natural-looking result, being also body hair, and requires no trimming. In one case I used both scalp hair and pubic hair at the periphery to mimic mother nature.

The donor strip from mid-occiput is excised and dissected to one- and two-hair grafts. The chest area is then outlined with marker as a rhomboid or triangle as agreed by the patient before surgery (Fig. 1). I usually stay medial to the nipple. The recipient area is anesthetized with 1% lidocaine and epinephrine as a ring block. The chest wall is avascular with minimal bleeding when compared to the scalp, so anesthesia may last up to 3 h after injection.

After injecting a small amount of tumescent fluid, incisions are premade at random using a 20 G needle for one-hair grafts and a 19 G needle for two-hair grafts. The angle should be flat as possible. Hair close to the neck should direct upward. Controlling the angle and direction, however, is not easy as the chest skin is comparatively thin. Moreover, the entire hair shaft, while sitting on a comparatively fat area, has the potential to sink into the dermis. At the end of the procedure one-hair grafts are stick and placed with a 21 G needle at the mid-sternum to contour density. I feather the borders again in a random fashion. From my limited experience, at least 1000 grafts of one- or two-hair follicles are required to satisfy the expectation of Orientals (Fig. 2).

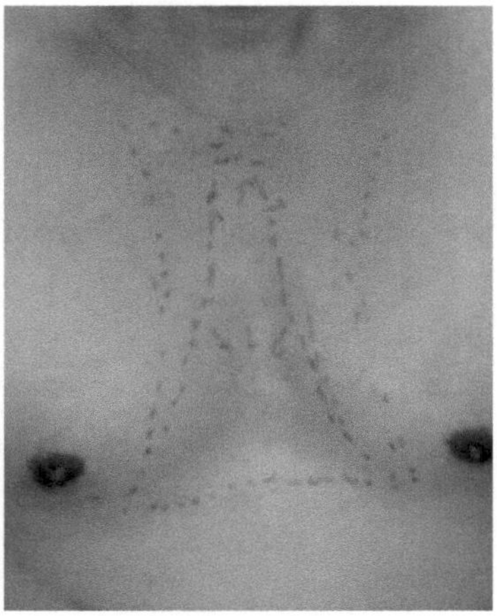

Fig. 1. Before picture in 1999

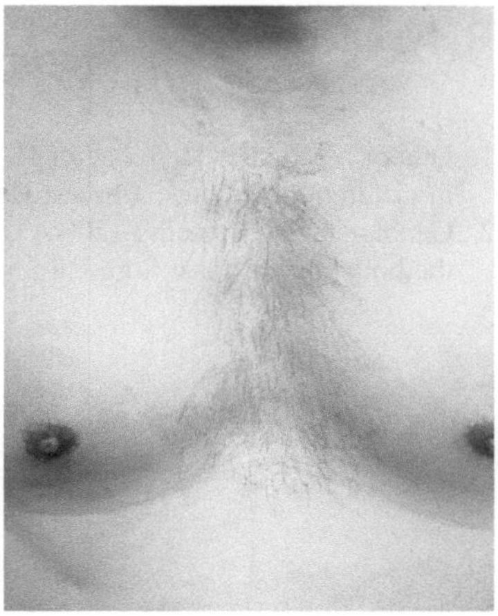

Fig. 2. Taken in 2008 after two sessions. The first session transplanted 333 one-hair grafts from the scalp and 161 one-hair and 195 two-hair grafts from the pubic area. In the second session, he had 105 one-hair grafts and 38 two-hair grafts in conjunction with sideburn and eyebrow transplantation. A total of 832 grafts were transplanted

Postoperative Care

Antibiotic ointment and a nonadhesive dressing (Melonin) are applied to the recipient area. One must be careful when the patient sits up after surgery, as the chest wall movement may make the grafts either pop or sink. Medical glue is recommended to immobilize the grafts. A short course of antibiotics and analgesics is prescribed before and after surgery.

The patient returns the next day for wound care. I advise the patient to be careful in the next few days in regard to moving the body and not to sleep prone. The grafts must be protected against rubbing for at least the first week. Carrying children (or other heavy items held against the body) is not allowed at least for the first 3 weeks. After that it would not be easy to dislodge the grafts by accident.

Sweating will keep the area moist and macerated; therefore, folliculitis and erythema are common after surgery as the covered wound is not exposed to air.

In contrast to a scalp hair transplant, most of the grafts will continue to grow hair without shedding [2]. The transplanted hair needs to be trimmed at least twice a month or when necessary.

References

1. Otberg N, Richter H, Schaefer H, et al (2004) Variations of hair follicle size and distribution in different body sites. J Invest Dermatol 122:14–19
2. Gandleman M, Epstein J (2004) Hair transplantation to the eyebrow, eyelash and other part of the body. Facial Plast Surg Clin N Am 12(2):253–261

Pubic Hair Transplant

S. Hwang

Hypotrichosis or atrichosis is a heterogeneous group of diseases with the majority being idiopathic (Fig. 1) [1–5]. These diseases, common in Mongolian women but rare in Caucasian women, often cause the patient psychological problems such as low self-esteem and consequent social withdrawal [6]. Surgical treatment may help the patient in recovering their mental health [7,8]. Before the surgical procedure, the patient's expectations and the transplant hairline design should be identified.

Because hair on the pubic area is composed of single-hair follicular units, single-hair transplantation is recommended. However, occipital scalp hair has not only single-hair follicular units but also abundant multi-hair follicular units as well. If we split the multi-hair follicular unit into single hairs, the survival rate decreases. Therefore, intact multi-follicular units are preferable to splitting the multi-hair follicular unit as they have a higher survival rate. However, three- or four-hair follicular units have the disadvantage of an unnatural appearance compared with the two-hair follicular unit. For this reason, single- or two-hair follicular units are used for pubic hair transplantation.

Method

Donor Preparation

Donor preparation is the same as with other hair transplantations such as with male pattern hair loss. We usually harvest a donor strip of 1000 to 1500 hairs. The next step is to create follicular unit grafts from the harvested donor tissue.

Anesthesia on the Recipient Site

For the pubic area, 1% lidocaine with 1:100000 epinephrine is sufficient. To reduce the pain during anesthesia, the sequence of lidocaine injection should be

D. Pathomvanich and K. Imagawa (eds.), *Hair Restoration Surgery in Asians*
DOI 10.1007/978-4-431-99659-0_46, © Springer 2010

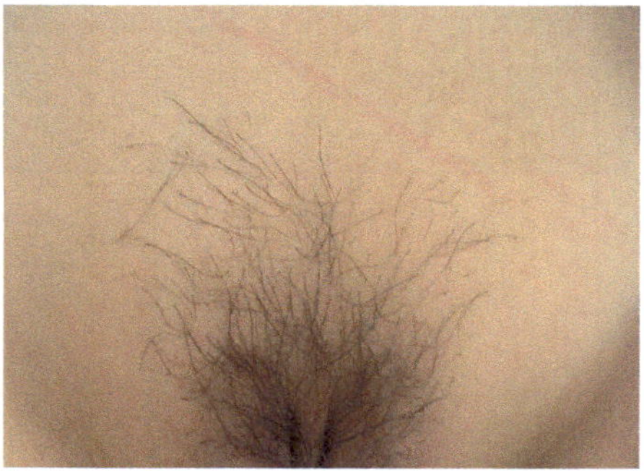

Fig. 1. Pubic hypotrichosis in a 26-year-old woman

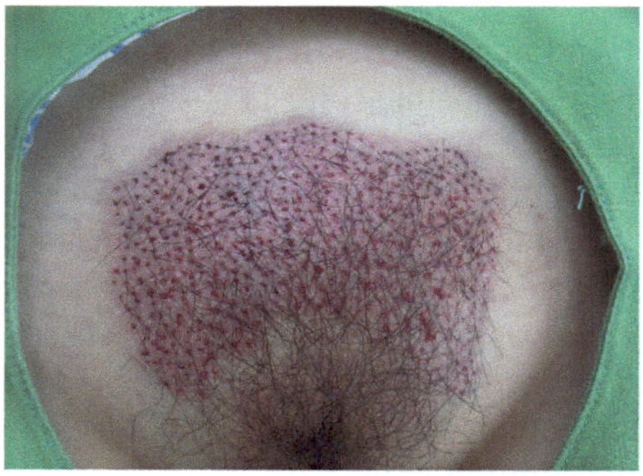

Fig. 2. Immediate postoperative state. Inverted triangular shape orientation of the hair growth is directed medial and inferior

administered to the periphery of the pubic area first and then to the medial area later.

Transplant to the Recipient Site

We can implant hair grafts into the hairless pubic area using the implanter or Western method. Before making a slit or injecting the needle, we can create a design according to the patient's needs. In general, a majority of patients favor the inverted triangular shape (Fig. 2) [9]. The orientation of the hair growth should be medial and inferior.

Personally, I choose to implant two-hair follicular units in the central area and single-hair follicular units in the peripheral area according to the design. It produces a much more natural result.

Postimplantation Management

The most common complication of pubic hair transplantation is poor survival (Fig. 3) and folliculitis and/or epidermal cysts (Fig. 4). The cause of this complica-

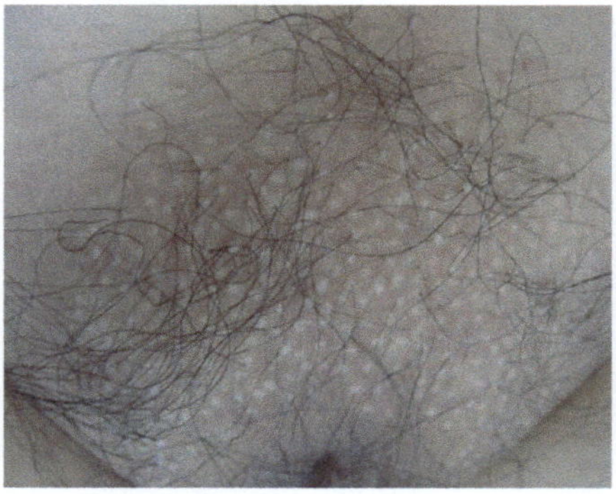

Fig. 3. Poor growth after pubic hair transplantation

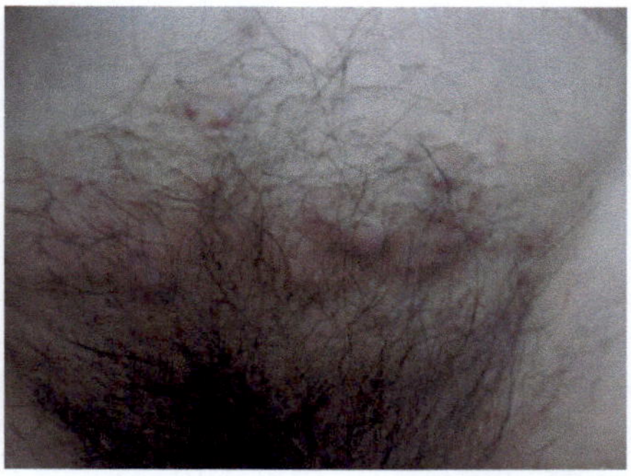

Fig. 4. Numerous folliculitis in pubic area

Fig. 5. Glue spray prevents the hair follicle from slipping down into the deep subcutaneous layer

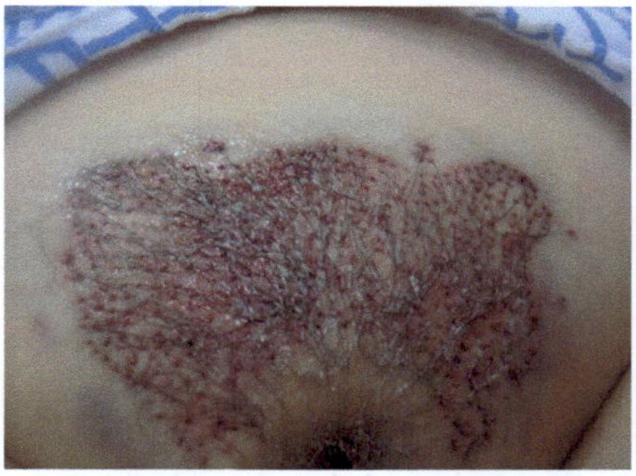

tion is definitely related to the seating of the follicle in the deep subcutaneous fat layer after implantation. Because the skin of the pubic area is composed of very thin dermis and abundant subcutaneous fat layers, the transplanted hair follicle is easily planted in a deep position of the subcutaneous layer. After implantation, some of the transplanted grafts are already located in the deep subcutaneous layer. To prevent this, we need to keep the hair grafts in a good position, without slipping down. My surgical advice is to prevent this by gluing the hairs together.

Personally, I prefer 3M glue spray. Before using glue spray, adjusting the graft level to the skin level is necessary. In addition, drying the recipient area with a hair dryer facilitates blood clotting. To reduce absorption of the glue into the wound surrounding the grafts, we need to wait for blood clot formation; this helps to reduce any sign of irritation or allergic contact dermatitis related to the glue. After spraying, the hairs stick to each other, which prevents the hair follicle from slipping down into the deep subcutaneous layer (Fig. 5). For effectiveness of this glue, hair at least 1.5 cm in length is required.

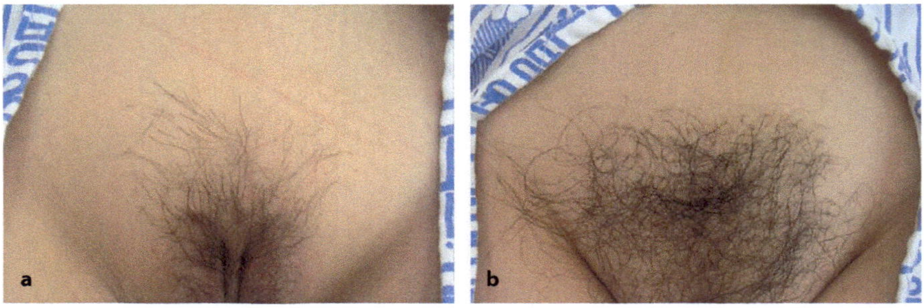

Fig. 6. **a** Before transplantation. **b** One year after 1,000 hair transplantation

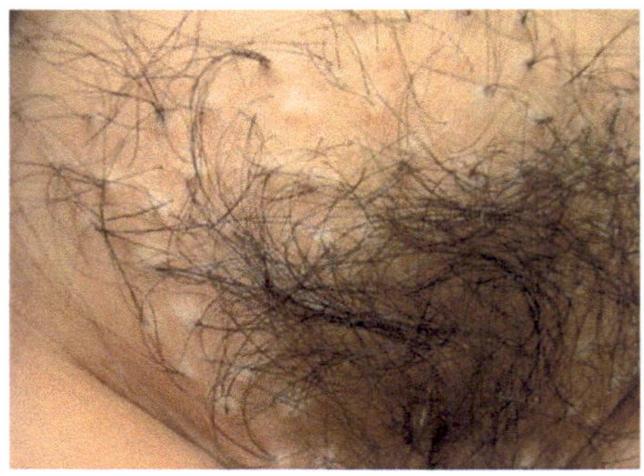

Fig. 7. Cobble stone appearance after mini-graft in pubic hypotrichosis

Long-Term Follow-Up

It must be noted that these hairs do not grow like donor scalp hairs. These transplanted hairs show only about half the normal growth rate compared with that of scalp hair, have a decreased anagen period, and grow curly on the pubic area [10]. Sometimes the patient does not even need to trim the hair as it will grow no longer than 12 cm (Fig. 6).

One complication of pubic hair transplantation is its unnatural appearance after the mini-graft (Fig. 7). It causes a cobblestone appearance in the pubic area, leading many patients to feel severe stress. Thus, the mini-graft or the three- or four-hair follicular unit hair transplantation technique is usually not recommended for Asian people who have very thick donor hair.

For a higher survival rate, the patient should be instructed not to do exercise such as running or engage in sex for 10 days after surgery, until the stitches on the donor area are removed.

Reference

1. Lee YR, Lee SJ, Kim JC, et al (2006) Hair restoration surgery in patients with pubic atrichosis or hypotrichosis: review of technique and clinical consideration of 507 cases. Dermatol Surg 32:1327–1335

2. Choi YC, Kim JC (2004) Pubic hair transplantation. In: Unger WP, Shapiro R (eds) Textbook of hair transplantation, 4th ed. Dekker, New York, pp 581–583
3. Jeon JY, Jeon IG (1982) The distribution of the patterns of pubic hair and axillary hair. J Korea Dermatol 20:231–237
4. Marshall WA, Tanner JM (1969) Variations in pattern of pubertal change in girls. Arch Dis Child 44:291–303
5. Marshall WA, Tanner JM (1970) Variations in pattern of pubertal change in boys. Arch Dis Child 45:13–23
6. Hamilton JB (1958) Age, sex and genetic factors in the regulation of hair growth in man: a comparison of Caucasian and Japanese populations. In: Montagna W, Ellis RA (eds) The biology of hair growth. Academic Press, New York, pp 399–433
7. Dupertuis CW, Atkinson WB, Elftman H (1945) Sex differences in pubic hair distribution. Hum Biol 17:137
8. Ignacio PL, Vicente P, Esteban GP (1979) The normal trichogram of pubic hair. Br J dermatol 101:441–444
9. Hwang SJ, Kim JC, Ryu HS, et al (2002) Does the recipient site influence the hair growth characteristics in hair transplantation? Dermatol Surg 28:795–799
10. Hong CK, Choi HG (1999) Hair restoration surgery in patients with hypotrichosis of the pubis: the reason and ideas for design. Dermatol Surg 25:475–479

Part XIII
Postoperative Care

Postoperative Care

J. Wong

Before the operation 500 mg keflex is given and again immediately postoperatively. Patients from out of town are given 500 mg keflex twice daily for 3 days. Immediately after surgery, an antibiotic ointment (mupirocine 2%) is applied to the recipient site and donor staples. We also provide six Tylenol 3 and two sleeping pills for the patient to use as required.

Patients are given verbal and written instruction to very gently wash grafted and stapled areas with warm water in the shower. The recipient area is air dried only; no towels are used for the first 4 days, after which the area may be patted dry. At no time during the first 10 days are they to rub the recipient area with a towel.

The donor area may be towel dried. If possible, patients are encouraged to return to the clinic for the first hair wash the next day and come back for a daily wash as often as they like until they feel comfortable doing it themselves.

Local patients come back to the clinic for staple removal in 8 to 10 days. Out-of-town patients are given a staple remover to have the staples removed after 9 to 12 days. After 7 to 8 days, they are instructed to soften the crusts in the recipient site and in the shower and gently rub off any loose crust with the fingers only, using no nails. They are warned about forehead swelling occurring the week following surgery and that the swelling may be quite bad, possibly involving the eyes. They are reassured that the swelling will be resolved spontaneously. They are instructed to avoid sunburn to the recipient area and to call the clinic if they suspect they might have an infection.

The patients are given a loose-fitting baseball cap to wear before leaving the clinic. Patients coming back for a daily hair wash do not need antibiotics. Occasionally, patients may develop a few pustules postoperatively; these will clear up spontaneously with an incision using a 25 G needle and gentle drainage using a curved forceps to expel the exudates.

There is no need for oral antibiotics as these incisions will heal very quickly. In 9 to 10 days, during staple removal most of the patients will request a short haircut so that the sides match the transplanted stubbles at the top. Asian skin with its darker tone does not show much redness postoperatively and looks very presentable after the crusting at the top is gone.

D. Pathomvanich and K. Imagawa (eds.), *Hair Restoration Surgery in Asians*
DOI 10.1007/978-4-431-99659-0_47, © Springer 2010

Patients with tight donor closures are warned about possible hair loss along the scar line and if it does happen to phone the office. Tightness in the donor site will relax after a few days, and any discomfort from the staples will resolve once they are removed.

The patients are contacted at 6 months to come back for a follow-up or to send 6-month photographs to our office.

Postoperative Instruction Sheet Used in Our Clinic

D. Pathomvanich

Your follow up visit after surgery is……………………………at………………………………
Hair restoration is a delicate procedure. Your adherence to the following instructions is essential for optimal results.

REMEMBER:
The hardest part of hair transplantation is waiting for the hair to grow. The hair transplanted today will not begin to grow until 3–4 months after the procedure. Before this time, small scabs will form around the grafts. These scabs will fall off in 7–10 days along with the shaft of the hair. **This is normal**; do not panic. The root remains behind. The new hair shaft will continue to grow underneath the skin, reaching the surface in 3–4 months. By around 10 months the hair will mature and add density to the areas. **It will take 10 months to actually see the result of surgery since the hair grows at an average rate of 1.5 cm per month.**

WARNING:

1. Do not drink alcohol for 48 hours after the surgery. Alcohol thins the blood and may cause bleeding.
2. DO NOT take aspirin, motrin, or naprosyn for 3 days after surgery as these can also thin the blood and cause bleeding (except when approved by your doctor). If in doubt, please feel free to call the clinic.

POSTURE: Do not bend over or lower your body to pick up things for the first 5 days to prevent swelling.

DIET: Do not overeat as this may cause stomach upset, especially when drugs were taken during surgery.

SLEEPING: Keep the head elevated with two pillows or a rolled towel put under your neck. This will help to relieve the discomfort of the donor wound.

D. Pathomvanich and K. Imagawa (eds.), *Hair Restoration Surgery in Asians*
DOI 10.1007/978-4-431-99659-0_48, © Springer 2010

POSTOPERATIVE MEDICATIONS:

A. An antibiotic will be routinely given to be taken before and for a few days after surgery to prevent infection. The new trend based on scientific research is to limit the course of the antibiotic to prevent drug resistance because the scalp is considered to be a clean area, except when you have an artificial implant (heart valve, total joint, etc.) The doctor will discuss this point with you before your surgery.

B. **TYLENOL WITH CODEINE** is a mild narcotic painkiller. You may take one to two pills, four times a day, **ONLY IF NEEDED**. This medication may cause drowsiness so caution should be taken. If you have to operate dangerous or mechanical equipment (car, sharp object, etc.), please inform the doctor for alternative pain medication.

SHAMPOO AND CLEANING:

The Transplant Area:

Your hair should be washed 24–48 hours after surgery. We want the graft to adhere solidly during this time.

1. Wet your head with a bowl of room temperature water or with a gentle stream of water from the shower.
   If you use the shower, block the stream with your hand so that the water pressure is not too strong.
2. Lather up the shampoo **on the palm of your hand**.
3. Pat this shampoo on the area gently (**DO NOT RUB**) and let it sit for 1–2 minutes.
4. Gently rinse off with a bowl of water, or a gentle stream of water from the shower.
5. Pat dry gently with towel. After 24 hours you can use a blow drier on **cool** setting only. **DO NOT RUB THE GRAFTS TO DRY THEM.**
6. Do this starting 48 hours after surgery, twice a day.
7. After 7 days you can begin to **gently** rub the grafts to help remove crusts.
8. After 10 days, you should be able to shampoo normally. However, scratching with nails should be avoided.
9. You can use any good-quality shampoo for hair washing.
10. A conditioner can be added to help in breaking down crusts.

The Sutured Area:

You can be more aggressive with the sutured area. Wash this daily starting 24 hours after surgery. However, please be careful about the knots that are located at each end of the incision.

NAUSEA/VOMITING:

This may occur after surgery, but in less than 10% of patients, due to the medication given during surgery. Do not panic because this condition is self limiting. Report to the doctor and he will give you medication for this. Only if vomiting is intractable would you need intravenous fluid.

HICCUPS:
This problem occurs occasionally and may last for 24 hours. Drink plenty of water at one time. Do not worry as this condition is self limiting.

BLEEDING:
On occasion slight bleeding may occur from one of the grafted sites, or at the sutured area. If this occurs just apply gentle but firm pressure to the area, using the gauze provided or a clean cloth. **APPLY THE PRESSURE FOR 15 MINUTES BY THE CLOCK**. The bleeding should stop: if it does not, please call us.

HEAD BAND:
This band should not be removed in the first 48 hours except when you are shampooing, or if the doctor tells you to do so. Continue to wear it for a minimum of 2–3 days after surgery. After that, it can be disregarded if there is no swelling around the eyes.

SWELLING:
On occasion, swelling may occur (in 5% of patients). It is not dangerous and is painless, and it will not affect the growth of the graft.

Currently we have incorporated anti-swelling medication in the local anesthetic. That is why most of our patients do not experience swelling, and even if it does occur, the swelling is very minimal. Applying ice on the forehead after surgery for 10 minutes four times a day will further decrease your chance of experiencing swelling.

DO NOT APPLY ICE DIRECTLY TO THE GRAFT SITE AS THIS MAY DAMAGE THE GRAFTS.
APPLY THE ICE TO THE FOREHEAD BELOW THE GRAFTS.

STITCHES:
Usually we apply two kinds of stitches. Your doctor will inform you after the surgery which type of stitches you have and what to do with them:

1. Absorbable stitches: there is no need to have them removed. It may take up to 3–4 weeks for the absorbable stitches to be dissolved or fragment off.
2. Nonabsorbable stitches: these should be removed in 5–7 days after the surgery. These can be removed by us or your local doctor. (Instruction sheet will be provided.)

EXERCISE AND ACTIVITY:
No exercise is allowed for 7 days after the procedure as this could result in increased swelling or lost grafts. After 7 days, mild exercise can be resumed.

After 10 days, normal exercise can be resumed.

SWIMMING AND SUN:
You should avoid swimming for at least a few weeks after surgery. **Remember acid, chlorine, and bacteria are in the pool!** After this, swimming is all right.

The skin of the grafts is not used to the sun and may burn easily. It is OK to go into the sun but with some protection like a hat to protect the sensitive grafts.

FOLLICULITIS AT THE GRAFT SITE:

On occasion, a patient may develop folliculitis at the grafted site. They are pimple-like lesions looking similar to acne. If this happens, apply moist warm soaks and antibiotic ointment to the areas three times a day. **PLEASE NOTIFY US IF THIS OCCURS AS WE MAY HAVE TO PRESCRIBE SPECIAL MEDICATION FOR THIS PROBLEM.**

CUT & DYE:

We advise not to cut or color the hair for at least 3–4 weeks after surgery.

SAUNA:

No sauna use is allowed for at least a few months.

GROOMING:

Hair gel, hair spray, and mousse are allowed for grooming 5 days after surgery.

GETTING INTO CARS:

Be careful when you get into a car! Make sure your head will not hit the rim of the door or the roof. Every year we have a few patients losing some graft from this kind of accident.

Part XIV
Complications

Complications and the Solutions

S. Hwang and K. Imagawa

For effective hair transplantation, we need to know not only how to produce good results, but also how to prevent surgical complications.

For each possible complication, I explain both the preventive methods as well as solutions, should these complications occur.

Nowadays, because we usually perform follicular unit transplantation, only complications related to follicular unit transplantation are discussed. These complications can be divided into two categories: medical and aesthetic.

Medical Complications

Undesirable Scar: Wide Scar, Hypertrophic Scar, and Keloid

Scarring is much more common in Asians than in Caucasians. Closure with little or no tension will leave a fine scar nearly every time. Tight donor closure can result in cosmetically unacceptable scars or necrosis (Figs. 1, 2).

To reduce wound tension in the donor area, the width of the harvesting strip should be less than 1.5 cm and less than 0.8 cm in the tight scalp. Occasionally, wide scars develop in younger patients, especially those with hyperelastic skin, even though there is no tension. In general, younger generations have a tendency to leave a larger scar than older patients, so be conservative in young patients under the age of 30. Trichophytic closure is also helpful to produce less noticeable scar lines in the donor area.

In case of a hypertrophic scar or keloid, a series of injections of intralesional corticosteroids (e.g., triamcinolone acetonide 5 to 20 mg/ml) is helpful to reduce the size or related symptom.

For subsequent donor harvest, it is recommended to take the second donor harvest about 5 or 10 mm apart from the previous scar rather than excise the strip including the previous scar. This is suggested because leaving two separate fine scars is better than a single wider donor scar. In addition, the width of the strip should be reduced to more than in the previous session so as not to put tension on the wound. If scar revision has been unsuccessful, W-plasty or follicular unit extraction (FUE) with implanting into the scar is another option.

D. Pathomvanich and K. Imagawa (eds.), *Hair Restoration Surgery in Asians*
DOI 10.1007/978-4-431-99659-0_49, © Springer 2010

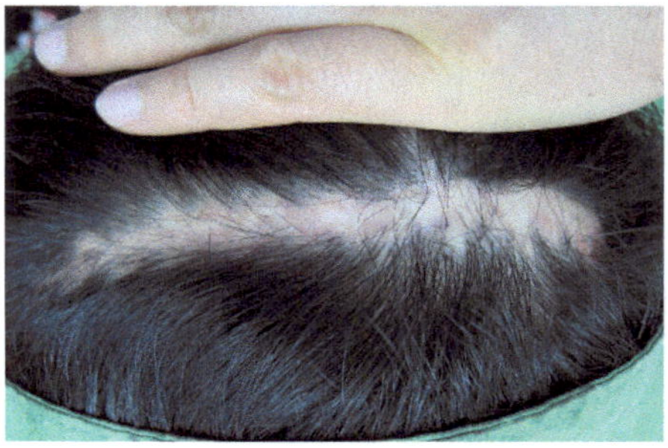

Fig. 1. Scar 2 cm wide on donor site of 28-year-old man

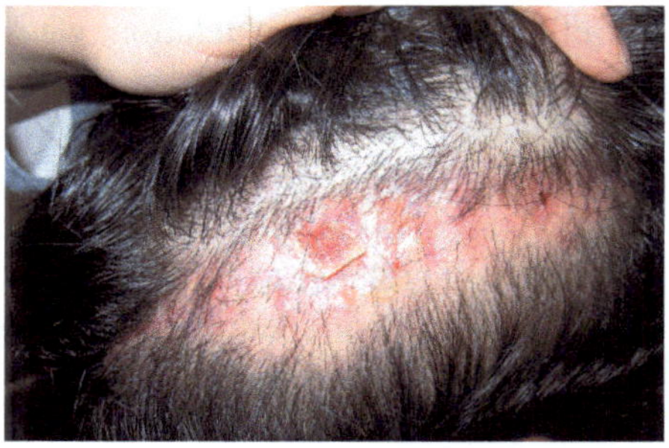

Fig. 2. Necrosis under excessive tension on donor area

Necrosis and Wound Dehiscence

When a wide donor strip exceeding the limits of tissue mobility is harvested, an extremely tight closure on the donor area will result. Excessive tension on the wound restricts circulation of blood, and it may result in necrosis and wound dehiscence. To prevent this from occurring, first reduce the wound width as much as possible and examine whether there is tension. If the closure is tension free, decide whether the strip can be widened a little bit more. Second, in case of too much tension on the wound after donor harvest, it is best to suture the wound as close as possible and leave the rest to heal by secondary intention. This method will produce a more acceptable scar and prevent necrosis.

Pain, Numbness, Hypoesthesia, Hyperesthesia, and Neuralgia

Pain or even anxiety about pain during operation can be minimized with adequate anesthesia and anxiolytics.

Most patients experience only mild pain in the donor area after surgery that can be controlled adequately by analgesics such as Tylenol. Many patients complain of numbness, hypoesthesia, or hyperesthesia on the donor or recipient site, but this usually disappears within several months after the surgery. Occasionally, some patients may experience neuralgia: a sharp, shooting pain or an uncomfortable burning or tingling sensation on the head, superior to the donor area.

Neuralgia may be the result of nerve injury in the donor area followed by abnormal nerve healing. It is helpful to inject corticosteroid mixed with 0.5% bupivacaine into the donor suture site. To reduce dysesthesia, (1) electrical coagulation is prohibited or minimized during surgery, (2) dissection should be done as superficially as possible in the subcutaneous fat layer to avoid damage to the neurovascular bundles in the deep layer, (3) and tension on the donor site is reduced for comfortable closure.

Folliculitis

Folliculitis can occur within 2 weeks to 4 months after surgery (Fig. 3). It usually disappears spontaneously in a few months, but occasionally a chronic recurrent form of folliculitis could develop. This may be caused by a foreign-body reaction of recipient dermis against the epidermal component of the transplanted hair or a small fragment of hair.

Fortunately, this problem eventually clears and rarely reduces eventual growth, although it can be delayed. Treatment consists of shampooing the scalp twice a day, antibiotics p.o. or topical, topical steroids, and drainage of pustules if necessary.

Infection

Infection is extremely rare in hair transplantation, but it can occur in immunocompromised patients with uncontrolled diabetes mellitus, liver cirrhosis (Fig. 4), or excessive tension on the donor site, among other conditions. As a means of

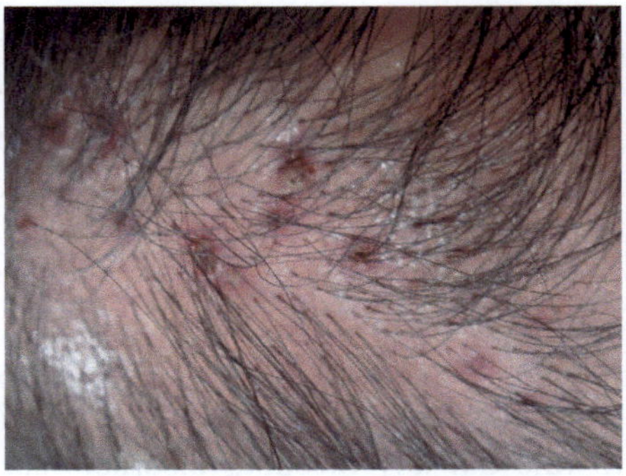

Fig. 3. Folliculitis after follicular unit transplantation

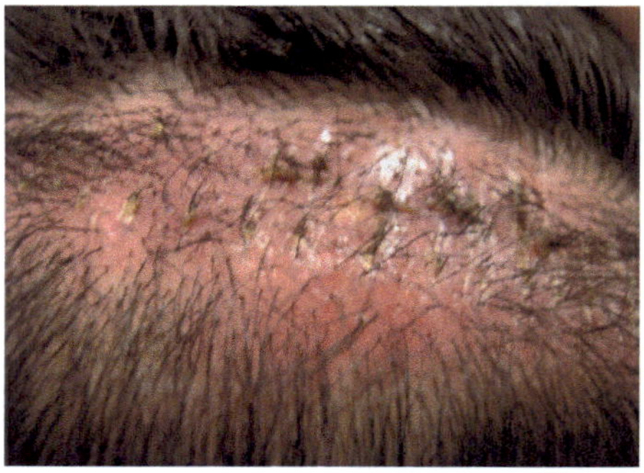

Fig. 4. Infection on donor area of early liver cirrhosis patient

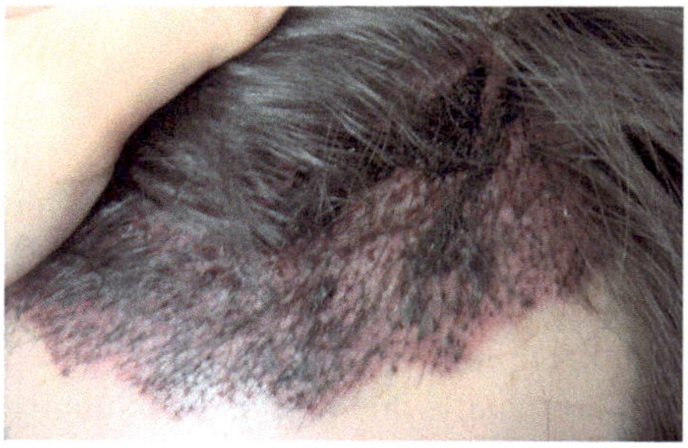

Fig. 5. Blood coagulopathy on the recipient area of patient with low platelet count

prevention, preoperative cleansing of the scalp with shampoo reduces the colony counts in the skin, resulting in less risk of infection.

The use of systemic antibiotics postoperatively is also necessary for prevention. It is definitely important to close the donor area without any tension. For treatment, systemic antibiotics are mandatory. The use of antiseptic shampoo such as surgical scrub is also appropriate for a few days after the operation.

Bleeding

It is very uncommon to see bleeding in hair transplantation. However, if patients do not discontinue medications such as aspirin and vitamin E for 2 to 3 weeks, bleeding complicates placement of grafts in the recipient sites (Fig. 5). Sometimes alcohol consumption before surgery and high blood pressure cause more bleeding in the scalp.

If there is bleeding in the donor area after suture, it can be controlled with additional sutures or an elastic bandage on the donor area. If bleeding occurs in the recipient area after trauma to the transplanted site, apply direct pressure with a gauze pad for 10 min. A blood coagulation test should be conducted before surgery to rule out any bleeding disorders such as Von Willebrand's disease, abnormal platelet count, etc.

Hiccups

Although very rare, hiccups may occur during or after the transplant procedure. Most hiccups are usually transient, but sometimes they can last 2 to 3 days. The etiology is not known, but it may be irritation of a sensory branch of the phrenic nerve that innervates the retroauricular area.

Hiccups have also been found to occur with the intravenous administration of diazepam or midazolam. In this case, diluting the diazepam and injecting it slowly is said to aid hiccup prevention. Treatment consists of lidocaine injection in the donor area, phrenic nerve massage, warm water intake, and medications such as chloropromazine, traquina, and simethicone.

Syncope

Syncope is uncommon but generally occurs when the patient stands up suddenly after lying down on the operating table for a long time. To prevent this, leg exercise, frequent position change during graft insertion, and frequent breaks with fluid intake during surgery are necessary. If syncope occurs, the patient should lie down again on the table. Then, vital signs should be taken and basic support given.

Aesthetic Complications

Unnatural Appearance: Unnatural Hairline, Bad Hair Direction

The hair diameter of Asians is much greater than that of Caucasians, so two- or three-hair follicular units make an unnatural hairline if transplanted in the anterior hairline zone (Fig. 6). Therefore, only single-hair follicular units should be transplanted in the anterior hairline area to achieve a natural appearance. The operation should be conducted by using the method that produces a natural hairline. Furthermore, hair should be transplanted in the same direction as the existing hair follicles to maintain consistency with hair direction.

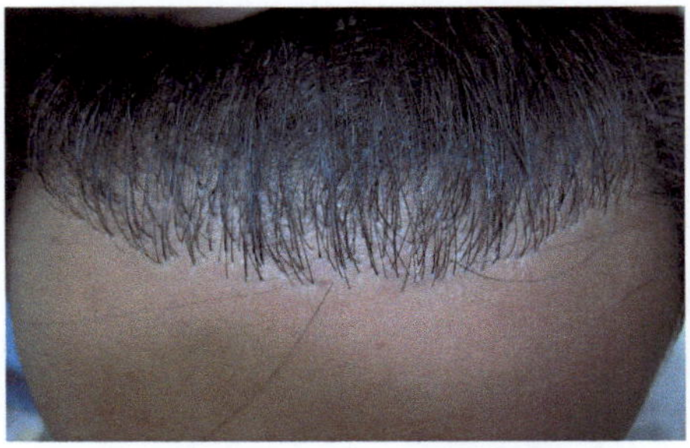

Fig. 6. Unnatural hairline after follicular unit transplantation

Poor Growth and Ongoing Hair Loss

Poor survival is also very rare in follicular unit transplantation by an experienced surgeon and assistants. It is caused by follicle trauma by mal-handling of the grafts during the procedure: transection, manipulation, desiccation, oxygen starvation, etc. To avoid poor growth, it is important to keep each step or protocol that may influence this result.

Even though the actual survival rate is excellent, growth may seem to be poor in individuals with fine hair (Fig. 7). Therefore, it is important to be careful when selecting patients with hair diameter less than 60 μm. Poor growth within 1 or more years after surgery occurs not only because of poor survival but also because of loss of preexisting hair (Fig. 8). Male or female pattern hair loss is not static but

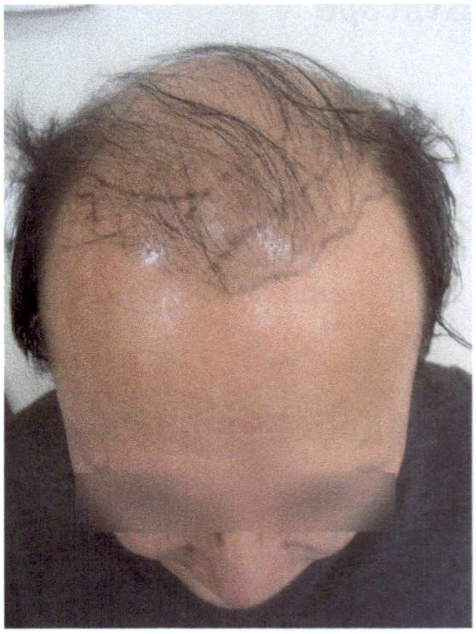

Fig. 7. Poor result in patient with fine hair

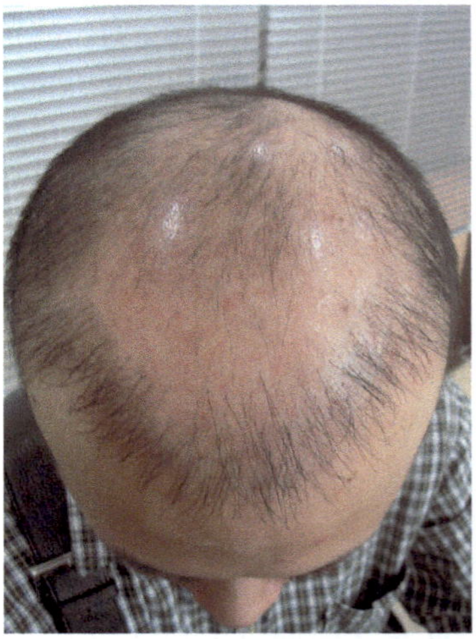

Fig. 8. Poor result due to ongoing hair loss in young patient

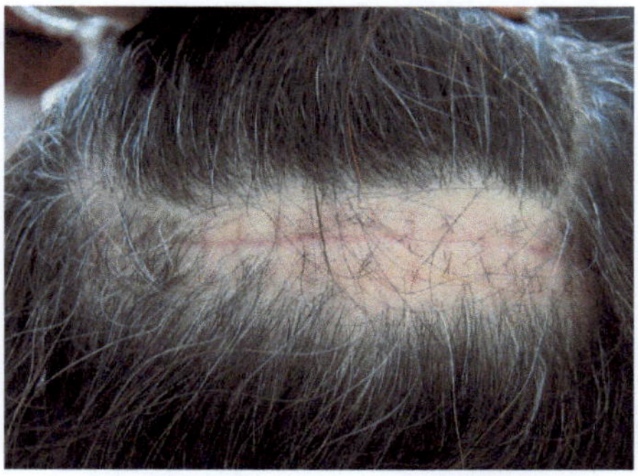

Fig. 9. Temporary hair loss on donor suture site

ongoing with time. Patients should be warned that hair loss is ongoing. If they are not informed of this, they will complain of poor results after a few years, especially young patients.

Therefore, medication such as finasteride is essential to delay ongoing hair loss. Sometimes use of hairpieces or heavy smoking affects the survival rate of the transplanted hairs.

Temporary Hair Loss After Surgery

Temporary loss of preexisting hair can occur in the donor and recipient area 2 to 3 weeks after the operation (Fig. 9). Regrowth of the hair appears at around the same time that the transplanted hair grows. Anagen hair can be shed along the suture line, possibly because of temporary poor blood circulation, which is especially more common in the high-tension suture area. Temporary hair loss varies from a small amount to a severe degree. Some of the preexisting hair follicles fall out because of poor circulation associated with capillary damage after needle insertion in the recipient area. It is not a complication but an inevitable, normal process if the patient has preexisting hairs in the recipient area. Shedding of preexisting hair is more common and more severe if the patient has more preexisting hairs that are more densely packed. Minoxidil use before and after the procedure seems to be helpful for temporary hair loss.

Facial Edema

Facial swelling prohibits patients from returning to their daily lives quickly after hair transplantation (Fig. 10). It begins on the second or third postoperative day and can last 3–7 days, gradually spreading downward from the forehead to the eyelids, nose, and cheeks as a consequence of lymphatic drainage and gravity.

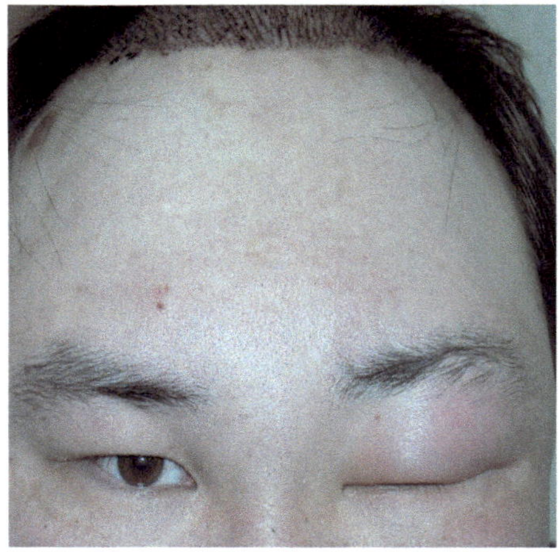

Fig. 10. Edema on forehead and upper eyelid at 4 days after surgery

It is severe in large sessions and in those patients who do not rest postoperatively. If it develops, there is no further treatment or medication available; therefore, prevention is crucial.

There are many methods to prevent or reduce forehead edema.

1. Steroid is the most powerful agent. It can be used in a mixed form in the local anesthetic solution or given i.m. and p.o. for a few days postoperatively.
2. Applying a pressure bandage or turban-style wrap is also helpful.
3. Ice packs on the forehead (not on the transplanted area) are beneficial.
4. Body positioning such as supine or lateral decubitus for 2 days after surgery helps the lymphatic drainage flow toward the temporal and occipital scalp because of gravity, resulting in no or minimal forehead edema.

S. Hwang

Pitting

There is also an upsurge of complaints concerning close-up defects such as pitting and tenting due to the higher expectation from patients.

"Pitting" is defined as the depressed appearance of the grafts as a result of implanting the hair follicle units deeper than the surrounding skin surface (Fig. 11). It is noticeable under direct light and is caused by these situations:

1. Slits and holes being too deep
2. Slits and holes being bigger than the grafts

Pitting used to be seen in conventional micro- and mini-grafting. (See Fig. 2 in chapter on "Omnigraft™").

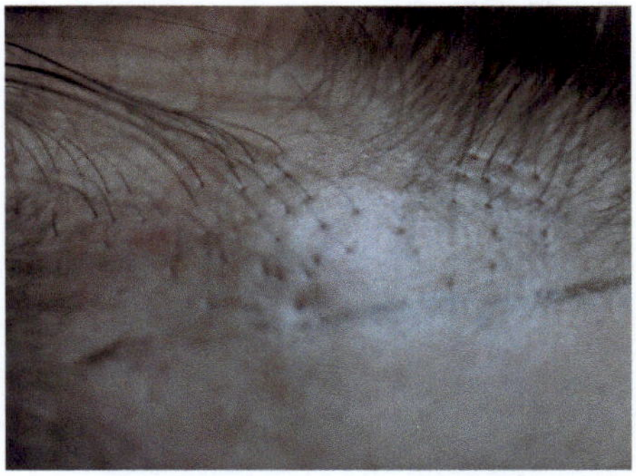

Fig. 11. Pitting

Prevention of Pitting

1. Make the slits and holes of appropriately the same size as the graft
2. Avoid the use of punch grafts
3. Avoid burying the grafts

Repair of Pitting

1. Adding on density by follicular unit transplantation can camouflage the pits. An additional session is expected as large quantities of grafts are usually required.
2. Excise the pitted grafts using a 1- to 1.2-mm punch in selected cases.
3. Use electro-epilation.

Tenting (Goosebump Appearance)

"Tenting" is defined as the elevated appearance of the grafts above the surrounding skin surface and is more noticeable under direct light. The causes of tenting remain a dilemma but are probably related to too-superficial placing of the grafts. Overgrowth of the epithelium during the healing process may also play a role (Fig. 12) [2].

Prevention of Tenting

It is impossible to predict the occurrence of tenting. The following precautions may help to minimize this condition.

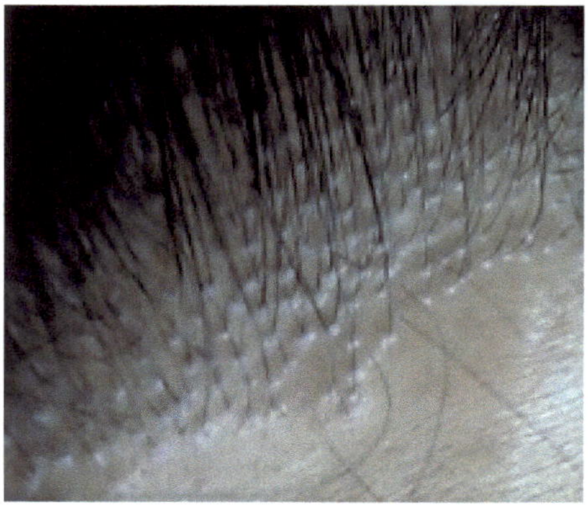

Fig. 12. Tenting

1. Create slits appropriately the same size as the grafts.
2. Check for graft elevation caused by popping-out or too-superficial planting at the end of the insertion and correct accordingly.
3. Attention must be given to cases with a large difference in the thickness between recipient and donor skin.
4. Make acute-angle incisions when placing the grafts into very thin recipient skin.

Correction of Tenting

1. Most cases will improve with time.
2. Add on density by follicular unit transplantation to camouflage the tents. The grafts should be placed deeper than in the previous session. An additional session is expected as a large quantity of grafts is usually required.
3. Any of the following can also be considered when tenting has not resolved with time:
   - Dermabrasion
   - Laser resurfacing
   - Electro-cautery
   - Topical steroid ointment of moderate potency
   - Low-dose steroid injection

K. Imagawa

References

1. Cooley JE (2005) Dilemmas in hair restoration. Hair Transplant Forum Int 15:207–208
2. Imagawa K (2008) Pitting and tenting. J Jpn Soc Aesthetic Reconstruct Surg 30:98–103 (in Japanese)

Part XV
The Business Side

Marketing and Management

K. Imagawa

With advancement in the surgical techniques, the public image of hair restoration surgery has greatly improved over the past two decades [1]. Nevertheless, such advances demand more meticulous effort in every single step, thus requiring increased time and labor. New hair surgeons, consequently, may find it difficult to start a practice in hair restoration.

Keeping up with the latest developments and learning the pearls from experienced surgeons are indispensable to attain and maintain competency, which requires continuous commitment to the following even after the clinic is set up:

- Attend academic conferences
- Attend workshops
- Train good staff members

Staff Training

In Japan and Korea, making incisions in the recipient site is the duty of the physician. The assistants are not allowed to perform the stick-and-place technique. The assistants should therefore be trained to take up other important roles in the recent trend of intensive laboring in mega-sessions.

Listed below is our scheduled timetable in training assistants.

1. Orientation tour in the practical workplace during an interview. A few candidates will withdraw their applications after the tour.
2. One-month basic training. New employees will attend general orientation for the first week. They are then assigned to graft preparation.
3. Participation in graft insertion. A few applicants will withdraw their application during this step.

Experienced staff will supervise the newcomers on a one-to-one basis during this training period and report their progress.

D. Pathomvanich and K. Imagawa (eds.), *Hair Restoration Surgery in Asians*
DOI 10.1007/978-4-431-99659-0_50, © Springer 2010

Marketing

According to the 2009 practice census of the International Society of Hair Restoration Surgery, the market for hair restoration has grown significantly in Asia: 78 822 procedures were performed in 2008 compared to 57 542 in 2006 [1].

While hair transplantation shares about 25% of the U.S. hair-related market, it accounted for only 2% in Japan in 2005. This figure includes artificial fiber implantation. I believe there remains great potential in the Japanese market [2,3].

Nevertheless, we have to take into consideration that medical advertising is much more restricted in most Asian countries than in the United States. Promotional information that is allowed to be disclosed and distributed is quite limited. Governed by this factor, it is rather difficult to stand out from competitors by using conventional media [4]; this is rather unfair as other hair-related service providers, when performing nonmedical procedures, can advertise freely. Fortunately, we have another channel for releasing our information: the Internet. Publicity on the Internet is simple when compared with other media. Advertisements can reach people globally. One major advantage of the Internet is that an enormous database can be transferred at high speed and received instantly by its users. Patients can have access to a wide range of information and even receive long-distance consultation without any geographic constraint [5–7].

Two successful examples of our Internet advertising are discussed here.

1. Real-time follow-up: this provides the viewers with the latest progress of a patient from before the procedure until months after when the result becomes evident. When compared with the conventional "before and after" gallery, it draws much more attention and hits on our website. We must however be prepared that sometimes the result may not be as expected.
2. Chat room: viewers can discuss their ideas or questions. At one stage, we had more than 10 000 contributors. Any positive opinion would obviously enhance our credibility. On the other hand, the physician's reputation can be destroyed simply by viewers' complaints or by being unable to provide answers to some difficult questions.

We should be aware of the downside of the Internet [8]. There is a lot of discussion and many forums comparing the different hair transplant surgeons. Most of the comments are untrue, including virulent slanders. We cannot and should not challenge all such incorrect comments [9,10]. Another problem with the Internet is the cost for listing. Although the advertising fee on the Internet is still rather low at present, it will surely increase in the very near future, as is evident by looking at the fierce competition for the paid columns in search engines such as Google and Overture [11].

The advertising costs in the use of traditional media such as yellow pages, magazines, signboards, radio, television, etc., are on the rise. In the United States, however, the competition among hair transplant clinics is so intense that the charge per graft drops year after year [12]. The discrepancy between income and expense has created a large burden for the independent hair transplant clinics.

Under these circumstances, it will become more difficult for those who cannot afford a huge investment to start or maintain a clinic. Small independent clinics will eventually merge with the large-sized franchised hair centers [13].

To avoid such happenings, we have to strive for a share in the growing market [14,15]. This aim can be achieved by these approaches:

1. Providing higher-quality work
2. Improving quality of service by all means
3. Advertising in an accurate and honest manner to build up rapport with the patients

References

1. International Society of Hair Restoration Surgery: 2009 Practice Census Results. Prepared by ISHRS in 2009
2. Kingsley S (2005) Solutions to solving the public perception of hair restoration. Hair Transplant Forum Int 15:9–10
3. Leonard RT (2006) Report from the Chair of the Media Relations Committee. Hair Transplant Forum Int 16:163–164
4. DiStefano MS (2005) Survey reveals hair-raising numbers. Hair Transplant Forum Int 15:194–195
5. Japanese Medical Law Code 205, 6-5, 6-6, 6-8, 73, and 74 (announced in 1945). A partial amendment of the Code: The items to which advertisements are permitted in medical practices (physician/dentist/midwife at clinic/hospital). Code 108. Announced in 2007 by Japan Ministry of Health and Labor, No. 108 (in Japanese)
6. Mangubat EA (2002) ISHRS website update. Hair Transplant Forum Int 12:141
7. Mangubat EA (2002) So you want to start your own website? Hair Transplant Forum Int 12:143
8. Manne F (2002) Internet tips. Hair Transplant Forum Int 12:139–140
9. Unger WP (2004) A commentary on internet websites related to hair loss and treatment. Hair Transplant Forum Int 14:17–24
10. Reed WH (2003) The independent internet marketing site: a symbiotic confederation? Hair Transplant Forum Int 13:255–256
11. ISHRS (2004) International Society of Hair Restoration Surgery: position paper on professionalism and the internet (October 15, 2003). Hair Transplant Forum Int 14:25–26
12. Bakhurin I (2003) Analyzing the effectiveness of your marketing campaign. Hair Transplant Forum Int 13:377–392
13. Rassman WR (2003) The future of hair transplantation. Hair Transplant Forum Int 13:419–428
14. Rassman WR (2006) The business of hair restoration: can new doctors penetrate it? Hair Transplant Forum Int 16:47–48
15. Puig C (2004) Growing the hair restoration market. Hair Transplant Forum Int 14:31–32

Part XVI
Hair Transplants in the Future

Hair Cloning and Follicular Cell Implantation

J.-C. Kim

The success of hair transplantation is often limited by the availability of donor hair. The use of donor hair from another individual is expected to be rejected without the use of immunosuppressants. Hair cloning has therefore been regarded as the future of hair transplantation.

Hair cloning is based on the inductive capacity of the dermal papilla cell to form a new hair follicle. This property of the dermal papilla is retained throughout adult life. It is important to note that epithelial cells must be present together with dermal papilla cells to form new hair follicles. Just one or the other cannot form a hair follicle on its own.

A few hair follicles are first excised from the occipital scalp by biopsy punch. These follicles are then dissected to isolate the dermal papilla. Each dermal papilla contains about 200–400 cells. These cells can be cultured in the laboratory to make several million offspring cells. Upon reinjection into the bald scalp of the same individual, the cultured dermal papilla cells will induce the development of new hair follicles. This process is basically hair multiplication or follicular neogenesis rather than true "cloning." The term "hair cloning" is therefore a misnomer.

With studies on rodents, many researchers showed that only dermal papilla cells are required for culture without the need for the epithelial component (Fig. 1). When injected into the scalp, the cultured cells will work with the local epithelial cells to induce new hair follicles.

Although the principle of hair cloning is proven, turning it into a practical technique for clinical use is full of problems.

1. The new hair follicles induced in studies using rodents are usually disorientated and grow at all sorts of angles.
2. In rodent studies, hair follicles induced by hair cloning do not have an even distribution over the skin as seen in natural hair follicles. Rather, they appear as clumps of growing hair (Fig. 2). The cosmetic appearance of this clumpy growth is generally unacceptable.
3. Once cloned hair was shed in the normal hair cycle, it did not follow the cycle and grow again. Normal hair grows in cycles that last 2 to 6 years, then sheds and lies dormant for about 3 months before the follicle produces a new hair and starts the hair cycle over again.

D. Pathomvanich and K. Imagawa (eds.), *Hair Restoration Surgery in Asians*
DOI 10.1007/978-4-431-99659-0_51,

Fig. 1. Hair cloning on mouse

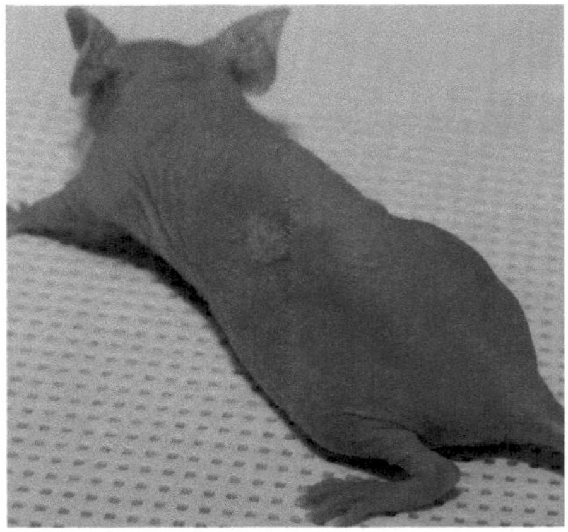

Fig. 2. Close-up view of cloned hair

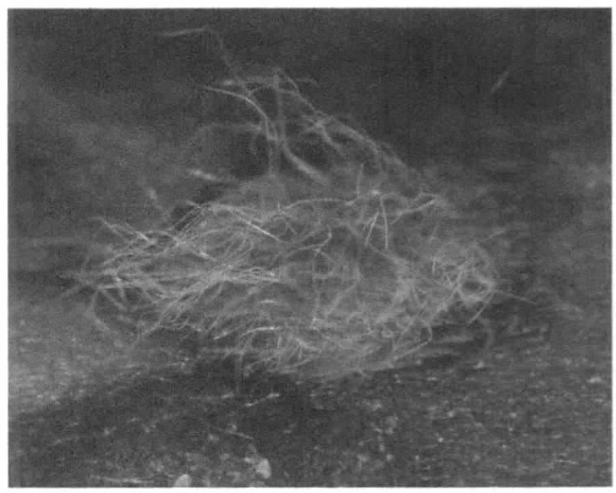

4. There is no study actually published to prove that hair cloning would work in humans. Although there have been unofficial reports about successful hair growth in humans induced by the use of cultured dermal papilla cells, the quoted success rate was unfortunately rather poor. A major technical problem to clone hair in humans is that cells in culture lose the ability to produce new hair, which appears to be the single greatest obstacle to this form of therapy coming to fruition. Finding the proper environment in which the cells can grow and maintain their ability to produce new hair is a major challenge to researchers.
5. There are safety concerns that cells that induce hair follicles to grow may also induce tumors.
6. Even when these obstacles are overcome, there are still the requirements of U.S. Food and Drug Administration (FDA) approval to further ensure safety as well as effectiveness.

In summary, for hair cloning to work, researchers need to be able to do the following:

1. Produce a consistent number of hair follicles for a given number of injected dermal papilla cells

2. Figure out how to control the angle at which the new follicles grow
3. Produce a consistent level of density over the treated area

Follicular Cell Implantation

The size of the dermal papilla is known to be directly correlated to the size of the hair follicle and the fiber produced. The dermal sheath also plays an active role in determining the size of the dermal papilla. Cells in the dermal sheath were previously thought to only play a minor role, mostly as physical support to the hair follicle. Recent study has however shown that cells multiply in the lower dermal sheath and then migrate into the dermal papilla at the start of anagen. At catagen, the cells migrate out again back into the dermal sheath. Therefore, both the dermal papilla and dermal sheath cells define the size of the hair fiber produced and how long that hair will stay in anagen.

Researchers took dermal papilla and dermal sheath cells, cultured them, and then injected them into normal mouse ears. Mouse ears are covered with tiny hair follicles that produce tiny hair fibers. Cultured dermal papilla and dermal sheath cells injected into a mouse ear modified natural hair follicles already present and yielded tufts of long hair growth 4 months after injection. The injected dermal papilla and dermal sheath cells migrated in and integrated themselves into the tiny natural hair follicles already present in the ears. The new cells had apparently altered the size and growth cycle of the tiny hair follicles to make them much bigger and to make them grow longer, which in turn produced bigger hair fibers.

This observation makes several important points in terms of using follicular cell implantation to treat male pattern baldness. If implanted cells can be integrated with resident hair follicles, then patients with male pattern baldness could be treated. Hair follicles in the process of miniaturization could be boosted with implanted cells to force them back into a full-sized, terminal growth state. By exploiting the resident hair follicle structures as a guide for the implanted cells, the problems of erratic follicle orientation and distribution over the skin, seen in hair cloning studies so far, could be resolved. The small, natural hair follicles would provide the distribution pattern and angle of orientation, while the injected dermal papilla and dermal sheath cells would contribute the characteristics of large, terminal hair follicles.

Unfortunately, there is also no study actually published to prove follicular cell implantation would work in humans. Although good progress has been made with hair cloning and follicular cell implantation, there is still more work to be done before hair cloning and follicular cell implantation can become routine procedures that yield consistent results in humans.

New Tools for Hair Transplants

J. Wong

This field never stands still and there are improvements made all the time. Although I have attended every ISHRS meeting since 1992, most of the practical and useful tips I have acquired have been from live workshops and observations at physicians' offices. If there is something new that I think will improve my work or make it easier, I'm usually the first one in line to try it. Occasionally we do find something that proves useful but the majority of the time the new tool ends up in the storage bin along with all the others that did not turn out to be useful. I limit my comments here to tools used for site preps and graft placement. Most of these tools are not new but for us they are still the best at what they do.

Despite that fact that it is prone to breakage and has a rust problem that is unresolved, this blade handle (Fig. 1) is ideal and works well with a slight modification. Tapering the nose (use a grinder) allows the blade to be held at more acute angles for temples and eyebrows. The slender nose provides good visibility, and the design is quick and easy to reload. The Tykocinski blade handle (A to Z Surgical) has a more slender nose and so far, this handle seems to be more durable than the Ellis handle. To date, we have not seen any breakage or rust problem with the Tykocinski handle and this may be the better handle.

The tools we currently use that may or may not be specific to hair are (1) Mantis microscope; (2) 815S forceps from Robbins Instruments; (3) custom blade cutter from Cutting Edge Surgical (Kimberly, BC); (4) recipient blade handle from Ellis Instruments; (5) Tykocinski handle from A to Z Surgical; (6) Personna single-edge prep blade for cutting into recipient blades; (7) Personna double-edge razor blades to dissect grafts; (8) finger bowls; and (9) #10 Personna scalpel blades for donor harvest.

D. Pathomvanich and K. Imagawa (eds.), *Hair Restoration Surgery in Asians*
DOI 10.1007/978-4-431-99659-0_52, © Springer 2010

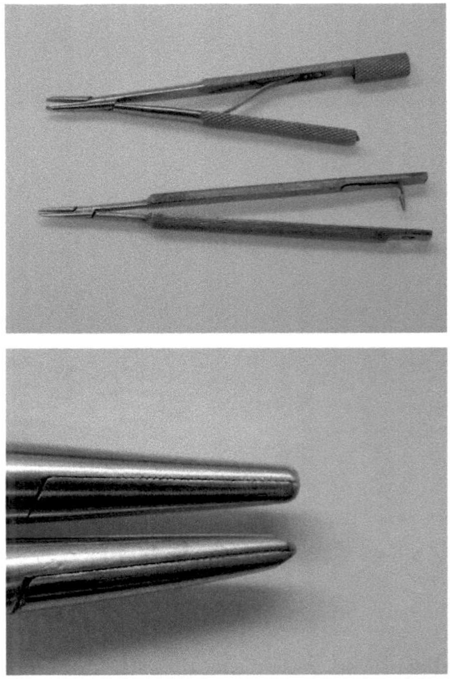

Fig. 1. Ellis and Tykocinski handle with modified tip

The major bottleneck with hair transplants is the insertion process. I have tried several devices, but no other than the human hand can insert grafts into these tiny slits we currently use. Some people are currently working on a robotic arm for graft insertion. Something like that is certainly on everyone's wish list. Innovations that truly work for graft insertions are pretty rare, but like everyone else I'm keeping my fingers crossed on this one.

Application of Stem Cells in Hair Restoration Surgery

D. Pathomvanich and R. Palakurthi

Stem cells have been sought for the treatment of various medical conditions, for facial rejuvenation, and for various anti-aging techniques [1]. Over the past decade many research centers have extracted stem cells from different parts of the human body such as placenta, bone marrow, whole blood, abdominal fat, and omentum.

Adipose-Derived Stem Cells: The Stromal Vascular Fraction (SVF)

These cells have the advantage over those from other sources as they have less potential to differentiate into undesired tissue and organs. Adipose tissue has been shown to contain adult mesenchymal stem cells that have therapeutic application in regenerative medicine. For scalp treatment, the focus is on isolation of the specific population or colony referred to as the stromal vascular fraction (SVF). This fraction contains not one but many types of cells, in conjunction supporting angiogenesis. There is evidence that adipose precursor cells have the ability to differentiate as well as de-differentiate into cells expressing a cardiomyocytic or endothelial phenotype as well as angiogenic and antiapoptotic growth factors [2]. Abdominal wall fat cells extracted by lipo-aspiration have been used in treating diabetes, coronary heart disease, stroke, etc. Success has been reported in the majority of cases [3–5].

Product Supplied: Kits

There are various commercial suppliers of adipose tissue products and devices, which range from large fat tissue-processing units to small benchtop devices. All involve a lipo-dissolve procedure and isolation/concentration of the stromal vascular fraction. For this study, we used kits containing a lipo-dissolve component and

D. Pathomvanich and K. Imagawa (eds.), *Hair Restoration Surgery in Asians*
DOI 10.1007/978-4-431-99659-0_53, © Springer 2010

an activation component (Adistem ADSC Kit A)*. The lipo-dissolve component is used to gently separate the stromal vascular fraction from the lipo-aspirate. The activation component is formulated to assist the cells to shift from a dormant state to an active state, which is measured by secretion levels of the cells. A standard benchtop centrifuge is required to perform the fat processing.

Adipose-Derived Stem Cells and Hair Restoration

There has been an unofficial report from Korea claiming success in using adipose stem cells to treat more than 30 cases of thinning hair. I had the opportunity in using stem cells to treat a total of five patients, including four male patients and one female patient. All presented with hair loss and were willing to try other modalities than surgery. The diagnosis and treated areas are summarized in Table 1.

The procedures were carried out on 18 October and 20 December 2008. These patients were selected from among a number of candidates as they were willing to return for a follow-up and to provide testimonials. Most importantly, they all retain some long and dense miniaturized hair at the top of the scalp. I was informed by the manufacturer that the stem cell technique will not work if there is no existing hair, and that it takes only 2 months to see the growth of new hair compared to 3 to 6 months after follicular unit transplantation.

Preoperative Preparation

Informed consents were obtained after explaining to each patient that stem cell therapy is a new treatment and that it may not work to their expectations in treating pattern baldness.

Table 1. Details of patients

Patient	Gender and age (years)	Diagnosis	Sites of injection
A	Male, 41	AGA Class VI	Front and top
B	Male, 62	AGA Class VI	Top, midscalp
C	Female, 36	FPHL, Ludwig II Thinning eyebrows	Top, eyebrow
D	Male, 42	AGA Class III Thinning eyebrows	Front, top, eyebrow
E	Male, 35	AGA Class VII Thinning eyebrows	Front, top, crown, eyebrow

*Details of the AdiStem ADSC Kit A can be obtained from their official website at http://adistem.com.

Each patient was prepared using the same protocol as in hair transplant surgery. All types of blood thinner products were forbidden at least 1 week before treatment. The scalp was cleansed with antiseptic shampoo, and a preoperative prophylactic antibiotic was prescribed. A test for human immunodeficiency virus (HIV) was performed as routine. Intravenous access was maintained using a 20 G cannula.

The patient was placed in the supine position and an area containing abundant vellus hair was selected and marked with gentian violet. An adjacent area similar in size and hair density was also marked; this serves as a control area where a diluted preparation would be injected. Hair density was counted using a Trico-scan and the images were recorded. At the selected area, hair was trimmed and kept for future reference. At the center of the primary test site, a 2-mm punch scalp biopsy was extracted.

Lipo-Aspiration

The lower abdomen was prepared with betadine and sterilely draped for lipo-aspiration.

About 120 ml tumescent fluid containing 0.1% lidocaine and epinephrine 1 : 100 000 was injected to the premarked lower abdominal area. A 2-mm multi-port cannula was inserted through a small stab wound just inferior to the umbilicus. A 10-ml hand syringe was used to aspirate fat cells with minimum negative pressure. Aspiration was stopped after 50 ml fat was obtained, and the syringes were placed in a bowl and left resting to isolate the fat layer (Fig. 1).

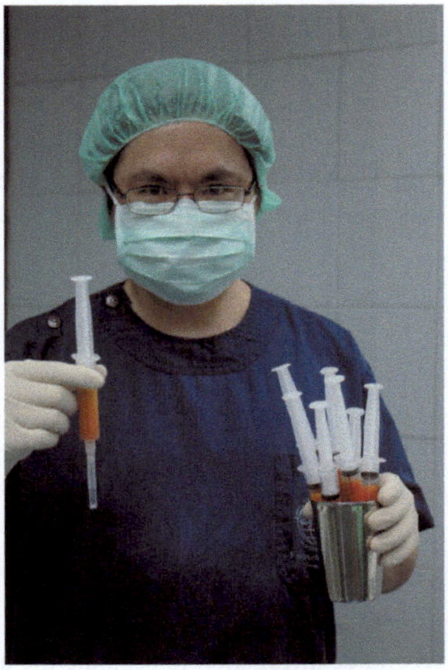

Fig. 1. The lipo-aspirate

Stem Cell Extraction: Isolation of the Stromal Vascular Fraction

The fluid in the syringes was discarded except for the fat cells, which were transferred to a sterile kidney basin and washed with the lipo-dissolve solution (Fig. 2). The fibrous tissue was removed to retain only the liquefied lipo-aspirate, which was then loaded into 10-ml conical sterile test tubes to centrifuge further at 1500 rpm/min for 5 min. Afterward, the fluid at the bottom of each test tube (below the aspirate) was aspirated with a 20 G spinal needle and collected into one large syringe (Fig. 3). After adding the activator, the pellets (now in solution) were let stand for 1 h.

The activator was subsequently removed by washing and centrifuging at 3000 rpm for 5 min (Fig. 4). The fluid that remained at the bottom of the test tubes,

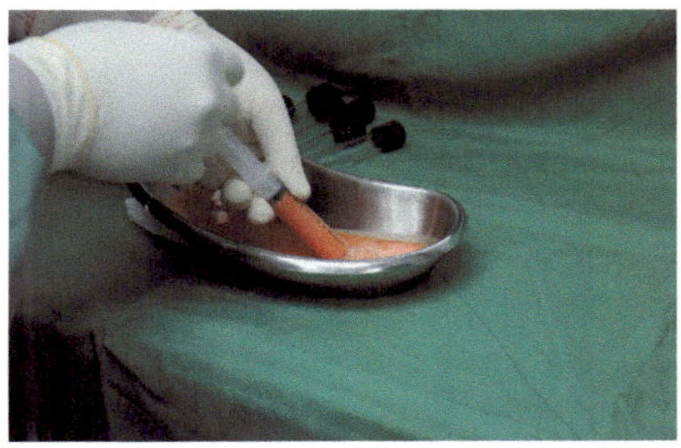

Fig. 2. Mixing lipo-aspirate with solvent to emulsify the fat

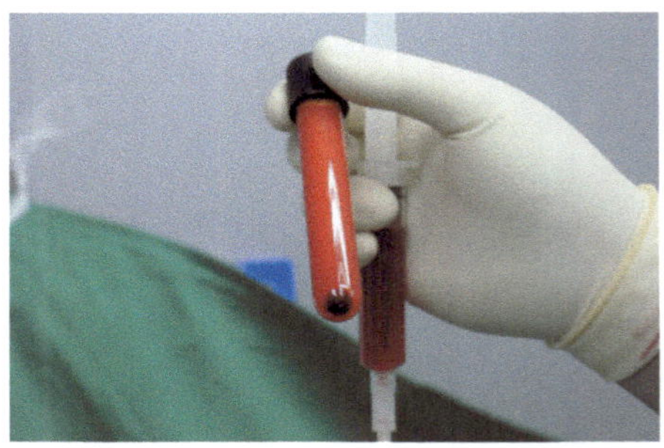

Fig. 3. After first centrifugation, the fat stem cell was suspended in the bottom of the tube

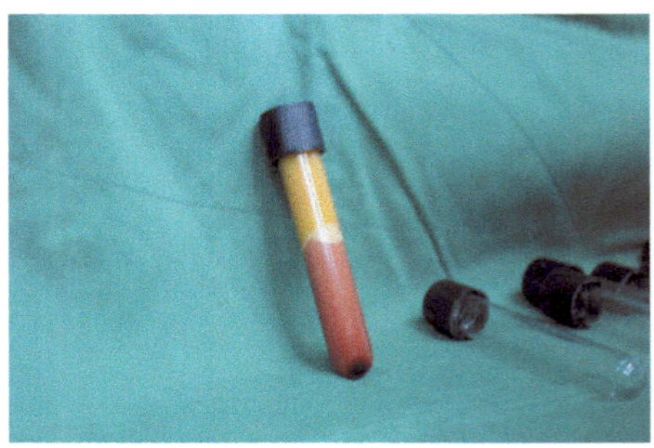

Fig. 4. Preparation was allowed to sit after second centrifugation to separate the activators

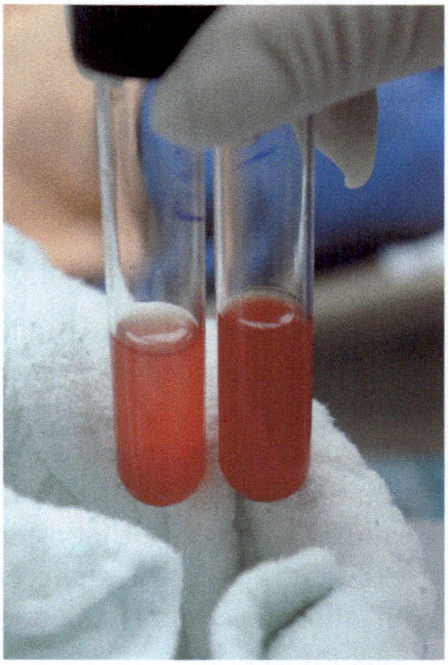

Fig. 5. Two preparations were prepared: full strength (*right*) and half strength (*left*)

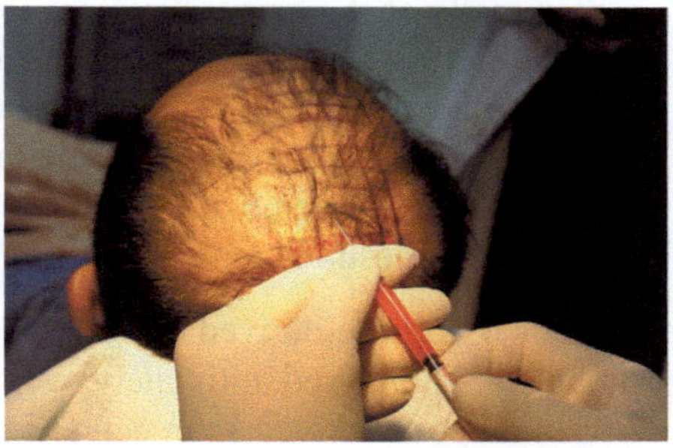

Fig. 6. Intradermal injection of activated stem cells into selected areas. The two preparations were injected into different areas to compare the result

which was expected to contain a small amount of SVF, was then removed and mixed with 5 ml normal saline ready for injection. In this case, it was decided to use full strength in one area and half strength in the other area (Fig. 5).

After the recipient area was prepared with betadine, a ring block was administered using 5 ml 1% lidocaine and epinephrine 1:100000 at each site. The 5 ml stem cell solution was subdivided (0.6 ml in 1-cc syringe) for ease of injection. Via a 27 G needle, the stem cells were injected intradermally, about 3–4 mm below the skin surface, where the bulge of the follicle is located; 0.1 ml was given per injection, 0.5–1 cm apart (Fig. 6). Two concentrations were prepared: 5 ml full-strength solution was injected into the anterior site and 5 ml half-strength solution, diluted with saline, was given to the posterior site.

Injection was completed without complications, and the patient tolerated the procedure well. All will be followed up weekly. So far no complication has been noted.

A 10-month follow up of five patients who had undergone adipose-derived stem cell treatment were disappointing. There has been no evidence of hair growth for both eyebrows and scalp hair. However, these observations were based on a single treatment of injections only. Further research is required to show if multiple sessions of injections done at specific time intervals such as every two months would show any benefits.

Conclusion

Stem cells have received significant attention as an ideal source of regenerative cells because of their multipotentiality and ability to replicate. The differentiating and de-differentiating properties of stem cells, with their potential for angiogenesis, arteriogenesis, cell preservation, anti-apoptosis, and anti-inflammation, open an unlimited future for their therapeutic use. In view of the abundance of adipose tissue, abdominal wall fat aspirate provides a definitive source of stem cells. The use of these autologous stem cells can prevent the many innate problems associated with allogeneic stem cell transplantation such as host immune responses and implant rejection.

Stem cells of the hair follicle are found in the bulge area of the pilosebaceous unit. Intradermal injection of activated adipose tissue-derived autologous stem cells may stimulate these stem cells to restore the normal hair cycle, changing the vellus hair back into terminal hair, or halt the process of miniaturization in areas programmed for androgenic alopecia.

However, questions remain to be answered:

1. Even if adipose-derived stem cells are effective, would the effect on the hair cycle be short lived, ultimately overrun by the genetic dominance toward AGA?
2. Will adipose-derived stem cells be helpful to increase the lost pigment cells in gray hair?
3. Can adipose-derived stem cells be used in other parts of the body with thinning hair such as eyebrows, eyelashes, mustache, sideburns, etc.?

Further research is required.

References

1. Park BS, Jang KA, Sung JH, et al (2008) Adipose-derived stem cells and their secretory factors as a promising therapy for skin aging. Dermatol Surg 34:1323–1326
2. Fraser JK, Schreiber R, Strem B, et al (2006) Plasticity of human adipose stem cells toward endothelial cells and cardiomyocytes. Nat Clin Pract Cardiovasc Med 3:S33–S37
3. Trivedi HL, Vanikar AV, Thakker U, et al (2008) Human adipose tissue-derived mesenchymal stem cells combined with hematopoietic stem cell transplantation synthesize insulin. Transplant Proc 40:1135–1139
4. Porada C, Zanjani E, Almeida-Porad G (2006) Adult mesenchymal stem cells: a pluripotent population with multiple applications Curr Stem Cell Res Ther 1:365–369
5. Reiser J, Zhang XY, Hemenway CS, et al (2005) Potential of mesenchymal stem cells in gene therapy approaches for inherited and acquired diseases. Expert Opin Biol Ther 5:1571–1584

Subject Index

MIX
Papier aus verantwortungsvollen Quellen
Paper from responsible sources
FSC® C105338

If you have any concerns about our products,
you can contact us on
ProductSafety@springernature.com

In case Publisher is established outside the EU,
the EU authorized representative is:
Springer Nature Customer Service Center GmbH
Europaplatz 3, 69115 Heidelberg, Germany

Printed by Libri Plureos GmbH
in Hamburg, Germany